Endometriosis, Infertility and Traditional Chinese Medicine

A LAYWOMAN'S GUIDE

Bob Flaws

BLUE POPPY PRESS, INC.
BOULDER, COLORADO

Published by:

BLUE POPPY PRESS, INC.
1775 LINDEN AVE.
BOULDER, CO 80304

First Edition, September, 1989
Fourth Printing, June, 1996

ISBN 0-936185-14-7

COMP Designation: Original work

Printed at C & M Press on recycled paper.

10 9 8 7 6 5 4

PREFACE

Endometriosis and female infertility are two women's problems which have gained wide attention in the mass media in the last few years. The incidence of endometriosis seems to be on the rise, if the media is to be believed. Likewise, since more women are attempting to have children in their late thirties, often for the first time, the incidence of female infertility also seems statistically to be on the rise.

Modern Western medicine's diagnosis and treatment of these two conditions is expensive, invasive, often iatrogenic, and also often ineffective. Traditional Chinese medicine, on the other hand, diagnoses these conditions without expensive lab procedures or invasive, traumatic operations. In addition, it also treats these two conditions humanely, holistically, inexpensively, and effectively. As Dr. Bruce Holbrook, in a lecture presented at the Third Annual Congress of the Canadian Association For Medical Anthropology, has said,

> Chinese medicine can cure most diseases that Western medicine treats surgically, with far less or non-traumatic techniques. A common example is acute appendicitis, the herbal-medicinal cure of which is a matter of course. Another is endometriosis—the Chinese medicinal curing of which should be sufficient, alone, to make the adoption of Chinese medicine in the West a Feminist issue.

As an American practitioner of traditional Chinese medicine specializing in gynecology, I am often called upon to treat these two conditions. Therefore, over the past ten years I have gained no little experience in dealing with them and the issues that surround them in our society. For some time I have felt that a great deal of unnecessary suffering could be avoided if more American women understood how these conditions arise according to the theories of Chinese medicine. If more women understood the Oriental causes of these conditions, they could themselves makes changes in their diet, exercise, and lifestyle to prevent these conditions or would seek out traditional Chinese medical care at the beginning when these conditions are still relatively easy to treat.

Unfortunately, too many American women first resort to the most heroic treatments of modern Western medicine. In my opinion, those treatments are better reserved for attempting to treat long-standing, advanced, and recalcitrant conditions more humane and gentle, safer and more natural therapies have not been able to cure. However, for this to happen, more American women need to know just how logical, sensible, and effective Chinese medicine is when it comes to treating endometriosis and infertility. I am confident that if more American women knew of the benefits and effectiveness of traditional Chinese medicine in dealing with these two conditions, more American women would resort to its use and, therefore, more American women would experience far less pain.

Because of this belief and my clinical experience substantiating it, I have written this introduction to the traditional Chinese medical diagnosis, prevention, and treatment of endometriosis and infertility especially for American laywomen. May it truly lead to understanding and, therefore, to prevention at best and early, easy, and effective treatment at worst. And may Chinese medicine come to be recognized as the universally valid, rational, mature, and professional medicine it is.

Bob Flaws, Dipl.Ac., Dipl.C.H., FNAAOM
August 1, 1989
Boulder, CO

TABLE OF CONTENTS

INTRODUCTION

Endometriosis and infertility are both professional allopathic disease categories listed in *The Merck Manual*, the "bible" of modern Western medicine.[1] However, although infertility is a traditional Chinese category of disease, endometriosis is not. This discrepancy underscores the fact that modern Western and traditional Chinese medicines are separate, different conceptual systems. Before American laywomen can understand the rational, sensible approach of Chinese medicine, they first need to understand at least some of these differences. This is because most of us Americans have been brought up on Western medicine. It is so much a part of our education and experience that we unconsciously tend to weigh, judge, and compare all statements concerning health and disease in the light of this dominant conceptual system.

The modern Western medical description of health and disease is not the only valid, logical, and systematic description possible. Just as a map is not identical to the terrain it attempts to describe, so any conceptual system is only one possible way of describing reality. Whether a system is a valid, i.e. pragmatically useful, description depends upon whether it is logical, self-consistent, and empirically provable *according to its own criteria of facticity*. Within a system, all concepts are relative only to other concepts *within that system*. The word system comes from the Greek *synistanai* and means to place together a group of things so as to create a unity or an organic whole. Because all systems are closed systems, one system cannot really be adequately described in the concepts of another, dissimilar system. The issue is not whether one system is more right than another but which system works better for the task at hand.

---

[1] *The Merck Manual of Diagnosis and Therapy*, Robert Berkow, ed., Merck, Sharp & Dohme Research Laboratories, Parkway, NY, 1977, p. 900

1

Traditional Chinese medicine as a system has developed over not less than two thousand, recorded years. It is a professional medicine, not a folk medicine. Its developers and practitioners have traditionally been the most literate and educated part of Chinese society.[2] Yet the Chinese medical system is based on a more general description of natural laws and events. Chinese have traditionally not separated the micro from the macrocosm. Although Chinese theories are framed in seemingly more general, what appear to a Westerner not to be technical terms, these concepts are precisely defined and logically consistent. In addition, they have proven themselves to be practical and empirically effective by more than a hundred generations of practitioners.

Therefore, the Western laywoman is asked at first to suspend her disbelief and not to try to assess the validity of Chinese medical concepts by comparing them to Western medical concepts. Some Western readers may say that these Western concepts are "facts", but in fact, they are no more or less factual than the Chinese concepts, since both sets are factual only in that they are self-consistent.

However, when trying to write about Chinese medicine in English we must use words which already have Western medical meanings and connotations. Therefore, the liver of Chinese medicine is not the liver of Western biology and whatever the reader may know about the Western liver needs to be held in abeyance when reading and thinking about the Chinese liver. If the Chinese liver is confused with the Western liver, then the Chinese concept appears quaint, simplistic, and archaic. However, when it is judged on its own merits within its own system, the Chinese liver is a very clear and practical concept illuminating much that in Western medicine is shrouded in the darkness.

I have chosen to write about endometriosis and infertility in the same book not just because these are two currently hot gynecological topics. Even in Western medicine, endometriosis may lead to or often is associated with female infertility. According to a 365 women study initiated by the Endometriosis Association of Milwaukee, 47% of the women surveyed with endometriosis

---

[2] Holbrook, Bruce, "Chinese Psycho-Social Medicine, Doctor and Dang-ki: An Inter-cultural Analysis", *Bulletin of the Institute of Ethnology*, Academia Sinica, No. 37, 1974, p. 97

were also infertile.[3] Among American women in their twenties, endometriosis is *the* leading cause of infertility.[4] Among the general American female population, endometriosis is the most common cause of infertility after fibroid tumors.[5] And it is estimated that endometriosis effects 15% of American women of reproductive age.[6] Even in Chinese medicine, the Oriental theories about the causation of both endometriosis and infertility overlap. If one first understands the traditional Chinese medical theory on the causation of endometriosis, one will be able to understand all the more easily the Chinese theory concerning infertility.

---

[3] Older, Julia, *Endometriosis*, Charles Scribner's Sons, NYC, 1984, p. 185

[4] Ibid., p. 8

[5] Ibid., p. 7

[6] Ibid., p. 19

ENDOMETRIOSIS

According to *The Merck Manual*, Western medicine defines endometriosis as, "The presence of endometrial tissue in abnormal locations, including the uterine wall, ovaries, or extragenital sites."[7] Julia Older further describes this condition from the perspective of Western medicine:

> In many women of reproductive age, some of the endometrial tissue ordinarily expelled from the body through menstruation travels outside the uterus and sticks there. In susceptible women, this tissue implants itself on the ovaries, the fallopian tubes, the outer wall of the uterus, the pelvic lining, the cervix, or the vagina. This condition is known as endometriosis.[8]

> Acting as though they were still in the uterus, these refugee endometrial cells respond every month to the same hormones produced during the menstrual cycle. So, although they are exiled from their uterine home, they thicken, enlarge, and bleed as if they were still inside the uterus. If the woman is lucky, these misplaced endometrial enclaves are not situated near nerve endings, and may not cause any pain at all. Otherwise, they can, and often do, make her life miserable.[9]

The first description of endometrial tissue found outside the uterus in Western medical literature comes from a French *surgeon*, Saviard, writing in 1696.[10] In 1860, a German doctor, Rokitansky, described endometrial tissue which

---

[7] *The Merck Manual*, op.cit., p. 7

[8] Older, op.cit., p. 5

[9] Ibid., p. 5

[10] Lauerson, Niels, H. & De Sevaan, Constance, *The Endometriosis Answer Book: New Hope, New Help*, Rawson Associates, NYC, 1988, p. 40

had infiltrated the body of the uterus.[11] This is called endometriosis interna or adenomyoma. In 1873, a systematic survey of this condition was done by another German doctor, Kundrat.[12] But it wasn't until 1922, when the American doctor, John Sampson, coined the word endometriosis and proposed a Western medical explanation for how endometrial tissue might get outside of the uterus.[13] Up until the introduction of the modern laparoscope to America in 1968[14], discovery of such misplaced endometrial tissue depended on intra-abdominal surgery, whether exploratory or corrective, and also on post-mortem autopsy. Until the adoption of the laparoscope, Western doctors had no way of seeing or feeling endometriosis unless the tissue had grown and proliferated so grossly as to be palpable during a bimanual pelvic exam.

A laparoscope is a fiber-optic instrument inserted surgically through the abdomen through which the doctor can see the insides of the abdomen. Through laparoscopy, a doctor can visually see misplaced endometrial tissue growing around the uterus, ovaries, or peritoneum. According to Julia Older, "Most doctors agree that the only sure way to tell if a woman has endometriosis is by combined endoscopy (visualization of the endometrial implants with a light-optic instrument) and biopsy."[15] Visualization usually means laparoscopy and biopsy usually means a laparotomy or the snipping of endometrial tissue through the same surgical incision through which the laparoscope is inserted. This explains the reason why endometriosis *seems* like a new disease.

Until people started doing post-mortem dissections and abdominal surgery, this situation *could not be known*. Its definition depends on the ability to visually peer inside the abdomen. When a relatively safe way of looking inside

---

[11] Older, op.cit., p. 171

[12] Ibid., p. 171

[13] Ibid., p. 8

[14] Ibid., p. 66

[15] Ibid., p. 48

6

the abdomen was developed (the laparoscope), the incidence of the diagnosis of this disease rose dramatically. In fact, we could say that this disease category is the product of the technology used to diagnose it. And that is exactly why this disease has gained increasing publicity since the introduction of the modern laparoscope to America in 1968. All the great flurry of professional essays and popular articles on endometriosis date from the 1970s.

At first, it appeared that endometriosis was a white woman's disease. Its diagnosis was mostly confined to upwardly mobile, white women in their late twenties and thirties, "ego-centric, career-oriented, (and) childless".[16] However, this initial assessment was a product of the fact that only the more prestigious and therefore more expensive MDs at first had the equipment to do laparoscopies and only financially well off women could afford such physicians. Those women, in turn, tended to be white, childless professionals. Now it is clear that the Western medical disease category endometriosis is "found in all races and amongst all socio-economic sectors of American society."[17] As Dr. Anne B. Ward states, "As laparoscopy becomes a more common procedure in developing countries, more endometriosis is being found."[18] This is an ironic twist to the Biblical adage, "Seek and ye shall find."

Endometriosis has been around since the dawn of recorded history.[19] It is just that the disease category of endometriosis is a relatively recently defined one in Western medicine. If we look at the accompanying signs and symptoms of endometriosis, we will see that all these complaints have been experienced by women for a long, long time. *The Merck Manual* states, "Endometriosis can be associated with pelvic pain, dysmenorrhea, hypermenorrhea, or polymenorrhea. Sterility, dyspareunia, and pressure symptoms may also be

---

[16] Ibid., p. xvi

[17] Ward, Anne B., quoted by Older, op.cit., p. xii

[18] Ibid., p. xiii

[19] The earliest recorded description of dysmenorrhea is in the Ebers Papyrus from ancient Egypt.

present."[20] In addition, endometriosis can also be associated with backache, painful defecation and/or rectal bleeding[21], premenstrual spotting[22], sciatica[23], urinary frequency, hematuria, dysuria, vomiting, abdominal pain, abdominal swelling, flank pain, and even hemoptysis.[24]

Dysmenorrhea means menstrual pain. Hypermenorrhea or menorrhagia means excessive menstrual bleeding. Polymenorrhea or shortened menstrual cycle means bleeding more often than once every twenty-eight days. Sterility in females is more frequently referred to as infertility. Dyspareunia is poking pain during sexual intercourse. Hematuria means blood in the urine. Dysuria means painful urination. And hemoptysis means coughing up blood. Pelvic pain means lower abdominal pain other than at menstruation. When this occurs at mid-cycle or ovulation, it is referred to as *mittelschmerz*. However, "The most common symptom of endometriosis is menstrual pain."[25]

In the same 365 women study mentioned in the introduction, 97% of the women experienced dysmenorrhea. Sixty-two percent experienced pain throughout their period. Fifty-nine percent experienced dyspareunia, 47% infertility, 68% diarrhea, painful bowel movements, and/or intestinal upset with their periods, and 41% nausea and stomach upset with their periods.[26] Dysmenorrhea is such a common symptom of endometriosis that Dr. Robert Greenblatt, Professor Emeritus of Endocrinology at the Medical College of

---

[20] *The Merck Manual*, op.cit., p. 900

[21] Older, op.cit., p. 29

[22] Ibid., p. 30

[23] Ibid., p. 30

[24] Ibid., p. 31

[25] Ibid., p. 35

[26] Ibid., p. 22

Georgia advises that, "every young woman with dysmenorrhea should be suspect (of endometriosis)."[27]

Although traditional Chinese medicine has no disease category endometriosis per se, it does recognize, categorize, and treat effectively *all* the signs and symptoms associated with endometriosis listed above. Chinese medicine has a differential diagnosis and disease mechanism theory for why a given woman might have one or more of these signs and symptoms. Although Western medicine has several theories about why endometrial cells may be found outside the endometrium (the lining of the uterus), they are all only theories, none of which have been proven as the conclusive etiology or cause. (*The Merck Manual* begs the question of cause completely by skipping any discussion of etiology altogether.[28]) Chinese medicine, on the other hand, can, in a logical and consistent manner, explain according to its own theories of physiology and pathogenesis why each of these signs and symptoms arise in a particular woman at a particular moment in time. And it can also treat each of these effectively and cost-efficiently.

Chinese Medicine's Theory of Menstruation

Traditional Chinese doctors base their diagnoses and theories on information gained from what are called the four methods of diagnosis. These include inspection or what the doctor can see with their unaided eyes; olfaction/-auscultation or what the doctor can smell with their nose and hear with their unaided ears; palpation or what they can feel with their hands on the outside of the body; and interrogation or questioning the patient about their condition and lifestyle. Inspection especially means inspecting the patient's tongue. Chinese medicine has a whole system of tongue diagnosis, the tongue being an internal organ which can be seen on the outside of the body. Questioning is restricted to only what a layperson knows about their condition. Lab reports are not germane information, and previously established Western medical

---

[27] Greenblatt, Robert, quoted by Older, op.cit., p. 185

[28] *The Merck Manual*, op.cit., p. 185

diagnoses must be considered with care since there is no tit for tat correspondance between a Western and a Chinese diagnosis. Palpation may mean abdominal palpation, but most importantly means palpation of the pulse at the radial artery at the wrist. Chinese doctors believe they can feel all the viscera and bowels, all the energy and substances, and in fact, all parts of the body by feeling the radial arteries at the wrists. This system of pulse diagnosis has been developed as a high art within Chinese medicine for not less than two thousand years.

It is from these sources that practitioners of Chinese medicine gather the information used to craft our theories of physiology and pathogenesis. Therefore, the Chinese style doctor knows only certain things about menstruation. First of all, we know that healthy menstruation occurs every twenty-eight days. We know it should be painless and accompanied by minimal pre and post menstrual signs and symptoms. We know the menstruate should be of sufficient volume, a rich, fresh color, and free from clots. We also know that the discharge should exit from only the vagina and nowhere else and should only last so long.

According to Chinese medical theory, the blood is created through the interaction of three viscera: the spleen, kidneys, and heart. The spleen takes the finest essence of food and drink and "sends" this up to the heart. The kidneys likewise send up to the heart some essence. *Jing* or essence is the most primal substance in the body. We are endowed with a certain amount of essence at birth and we also manufacture some from the surplus of energy we don't use day to day. Both congenital and acquired essences are stored in the kidneys. When the body needs either a quick infusion of energy or the substrate for building new tissue or substance, essence is used. Therefore, the Chinese concept of blood is created out of the finest essence of food and drink transformed and transported up to the heart by the spleen and from kidney essence. The heart combines these to create blood which the heart then pumps out to the rest of the body.

Menstrual blood is, in a sense, excess blood. It is sent down to the uterus by the heart in order to become the source and sustenance of the fetus. Since the Chinese did not use microscopic inspection, traditional Chinese doctors did not know about eggs. They could see the blood issuing from the vagina and babies too. And they knew men ejaculated sperm into the vagina and that only then did women become pregnant. So throughout Asia it is traditionally believed that the fetus is conceived out of the combination of the woman's blood and the man's sperm. For a woman to either menstruate or conceive, she must have a superabundance of blood beyond what is necessary for her own day to day survival.

The *Nei Jing (Inner Classic)*, the oldest written classic of Chinese medicine, says that women begin to menstruate at fourteen when their kidneys and their digestion, *i.e.,* their spleens, have matured, thus creating a monthly superabundance of blood. According to this view, until fourteen, women's metabolism is not mature and thus does not make sufficient blood for there to be enough to periodically brim over. The onset of menstruation both at menarche and each month is called the arrival of the *tian gui* or heavenly water.

In a sense, the uterus is like a cup. Blood is sent down to the uterus by the heart. When the blood collects sufficiently, it overflows and there is menstruation or the discharge of blood from the uterus. In Chinese medicine, the uterus and the liver are closely related. The uterus is the blood chamber but it is the liver which "stores" the blood. That is one of the liver's main Chinese medical functions. If the liver stores properly adequate blood, menstruation occurs on schedule and is normal in volume.

Another function of the liver is to maintain patency or free flow of the qi or vital energy of the body. The qi and blood are intimately connected. The qi moves the blood and so is its "commander". But the blood is the root of the qi and so is its "mother". If the qi does not flow smoothly, neither will the blood. In that case, the blood will not be able to overflow the uterus at the proper time nor in the proper amount. In Chinese medicine there is a famous dictum, *tong ze bu tong, bu tong ze tong.* This means if there is free flow, there is no pain; if there is pain, there is no free flow. Dysmenorrhea is pain during menstruation. Therefore, dysmenorrhea is lack of free flow of the menstrual blood and this is often due to the liver's loss of maintaining the qi and blood's patency. Although the Western anatomical liver is located below the ribs, the Chinese liver is "placed" in the lower burner or pelvic cavity. It is responsible for maintaining the free flow of qi and therefore blood in all the viscera and bowels located in the pelvis. In Chinese medicine, this includes the intestines and the bladder besides the liver itself and the uterus.

11

Chinese medicine believes that there are certain discrete flows of energy or qi which run through the body. These are called *jing luo* or channels and network vessels but are also often referred to as meridians in English. In particular, the liver, spleen, and kidney channels run through the pelvis and all can effect menstruation. Also there are three so-called extraordinary vessels which run through the pelvis and have a special effect on menstruation, conception, and gestation. These are the *ren mai* or conception vessel, the *chong mai* or penetrating vessel, and the *du mai* or the governing vessel. Especially the conception and penetrating vessels are said to regulate menstruation. The conception vessel carries mostly qi and the penetrating vessel carries mostly blood. The penetrating vessel is also known as the sea of blood and its function is closely connected with the liver. If any of these vessels is blocked, congested, or deficient, this will usually manifest in women as some sort of menstrual problem.

A normal menstrual cycle should span twenty-eight days. Twenty-eight days is also the length of the moon cycle. Therefore, in Chinese, menstruation is called *yue jing* or moon flow. This twenty-eight day cycle is divided into four seven day segments. The first seven day segment begins with the onset of menstruation and is the menstruation itself. During the menstruation, the qi or energy mobilizes the blood for discharge from the uterus and ultimately from the body. The second seven day segment is the postmentruum. During this time, the blood is relatively deficient, its surplus having been discharged, and the body is actively engaged in replacing this lost blood. At the same time, the qi in the body is traveling upwards and outwards away from the pelvis. It is at this point that the spleen is sending up the liquids to be transformed into blood in and by the heart. The third segment corresponds to the mid-cycle. At this point, the blood is relatively full and the qi starts traveling back down and in, carrying the blood towards the pelvis. The fourth segment of the cycle is the premenstruum. Here the qi is attempting to move the blood to the uterus in preparation for discharge. At this point, the qi and blood are at their maximum volume in the pelvis. Figures 1 and 2 show the important energetic relationships during the four phases of this cycle.

Figure 1: Blood during the four phases of a woman's monthly cycle

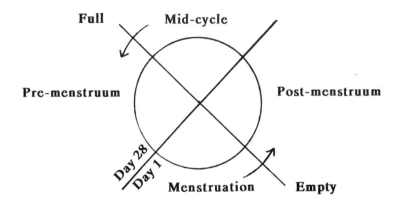

Figure 2: Qi during the four phases of a woman's monthly cycle

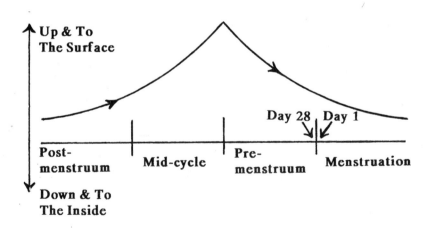

To summarize the above, from the end of menstruation through mid-cycle, the blood grows in volume. From mid-cycle through menstruation, the blood flows down and eventually out of the body. The qi, on the other hand, flows up and to the exterior surface of the body from the end of menstruation to mid-cycle. From mid-cycle through menstruation, the qi flows down and in, collecting and then mobilizing the blood. Because the qi and blood are a yin/yang pair, they are interdependent and their growth and flow depend on each other.

The Chinese Theory on the Cause of Menstrual Problems

Blood Vacuity

Based on the above general theories concerning menstruation, menstrual problems arise when some irregularity or imbalance occurs *vis à vis* the above functions. First of all, there may not be enough blood collected in the uterus to flow over as the menstruate. If there is not enough blood, this, in turn, can be due to either faulty production, over-consumption, or loss.

As mentioned above, blood is produced in Chinese medicine by the heart, spleen, and kidneys. If any of these three viscera are weak or vacuous, sufficient blood may not be produced. The spleen's role in blood production is paramount. Blood is primarily transformed from the nutritive essence extracted from foods and liquids through digestion. The spleen/stomach as a functional unit is the basis of digestion. If spleen function is impaired or deficient, adequate blood cannot be made. Mostly, spleen function is dependent upon right diet and proper eating habits. However, the spleen can also be affected by emotions, especially worry. Secondly, if the kidney essence is depleted, it cannot provide the initial substrate for the creation of the blood. Kidney essence is naturally consumed by the process of living, but stress, excessive sex, recreational drugs, excessive activity including mental and sensory activity, prolonged fatigue, coffee, alcohol, and chronic disease all prematurely exhaust the essence. The heart's part in blood creation is not so easily explained. The heart is the palace of the *shen* or spirit, *i.e.*, the consciousness. Any emotional excess can disturb the *shen* and therefore impede proper creation of the blood. Therefore, anything which impairs the functioning of these three Chinese organs may also impair blood production.

14

Blood's function, according to Chinese medicine, is to nourish the viscera and bowels and the body tissues. Therefore, it also is consumed in the act of living just as is the essence. However, if the body becomes overheated, either due to fever, inflammation, or hyperactivity, the blood can be exhausted or evaporated all the more quickly. This then leads to blood vacuity even though its production proceeds apace. Blood is part of the yin substance of the body. It is intimately related, therefore, to the other yin substances, essence and fluids. If either essence or fluids are lost or consumed, blood will likewise become exhausted.

Blood can be lost due to hemorrhage in turn due to traumatic injury or due to internal dysfunction. Hematuria (bleeding with urination), hemafaecia (bleeding with defecation), epistaxis (nosebleed), hemoptysis (coughing blood), and hematemesis (vomiting blood), can all deplete the blood so that there is not enough left for menstruation. Also, profuse sweating, protracted vomiting, or excessive dysentery and diarrhea can all lead to blood vacuity due to loss of body fluids in general.

For whatever reason, if there is not enough blood, this may lead to hypomenorrhea, scanty menstruation, delayed period or lengthened cycle, dysmenorrhea, amenorrhea, infertility, low back pain, dizziness, insomnia, anxiety, palpitations, and miscarriage.

Stagnant Qi & Static Blood

The qi moves the blood. If the qi moves, the blood moves. If the qi stops, the blood stops. The blood cannot propel itself. This means that if the qi becomes sluggish or stuck, the blood will likewise become static. The qi can become sluggish or stuck due to emotional stuckness or stress. Emotions are our subjective experience of the flow of qi. Qi and emotions are not two separate things. In our stressed out, modern Western society, emotional stress is the single most important cause of stagnant qi. Since it is the liver's job to maintain the free flow and patency of the qi, stagnant qi is usually associated with liver depression. Since the liver is so intimately associated with the menstrual cycle, liver depression and stagnant qi in women almost always manifests as some menstrually related problem.

15

In particular, stagnant qi most often manifests as pain and distention. Stagnant qi pain is dull, crampy, or colicky. It may shift locations or come and go in waves or is relatively generalized. Liver depression and qi stagnation may manifest as pain and distention, then, in any area of the body associated with the liver or traversed by the liver channel. Figure 3 shows the typical areas effected by liver depression and qi stagnation.

Static blood may be caused by either long-term qi stagnation or directly by traumatic injury, including surgery. Its characteristic is localized, fixed, sharp, stabbing or lancinating pain. Static blood may also be evidenced by bleeding, ecchymoses and petechiae, and blood clots. When blood stasis causes bleeding, it is because the forces the blood stasis forces the blood out of its bounds or normal pathways. Ecchymoses and petechiae are black and blue spots which may appear anywhere on the body. Clots mean that any bleeding observed appears clotty. Blood stasis due to stagnant qi in turn due to liver dysfunction may also manifest in any area of the body associated with the liver or traversed by the liver channel. In addition, blood stasis may be caused by any other of the so-called six depressions (which we will discuss below) and by cold. Cold has a tendency to congeal the blood and therefore blood stasis may arise due to such congelation. Women's pelvis and uterus are particularly susceptible to blood stasis due to cold congelation. If blood stasis is caused by something other than stagnant qi, eventually it will tend to also cause stagnant qi due to the reciprocal relationship between the qi and the blood.

If, for whatever reason, the qi and blood become static and stagnant, this can cause delayed periods, irregular periods, scanty periods, painful periods, periods which start and stop, abdominal distention, intestinal and stomach upset, sciatica, abdominal pain, flank pain, dysuria, painful defecation, painful intercourse, infertility, and painful labor.

Counterflow qi is a subcategory of stagnant qi. Qi is yang and therefore is warm and also tends to rise. When qi accumulates abnormally somewhere in the body due to blockage, it tends to float upwards just like a balloon. When it flushes up, it is called counterflow qi. Since the qi also carries or propels the blood, this may lead to various hemorrhagic disorders. In particular, pre or menstrual vomiting, premenstrual headaches, premenstrual breast distention and pain, perimenstrual epistaxis and hemoptysis are all due, in Chinese medicine, to stagnant qi which is vented up rebelliously.

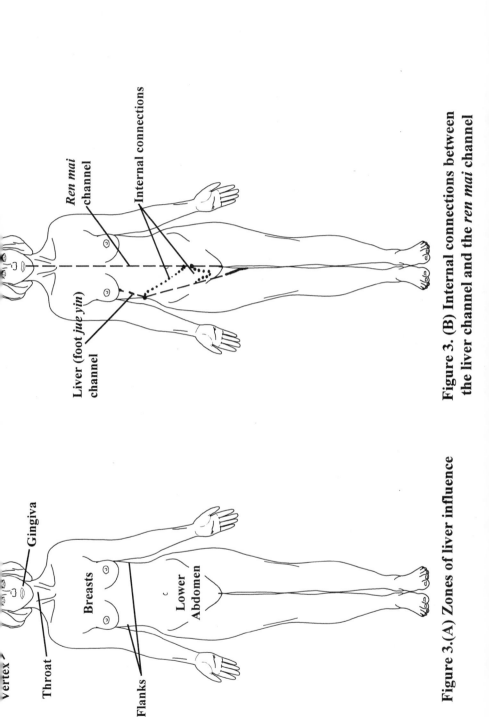

Figure 3.(A) Zones of liver influence

Figure 3. (B) Internal connections between the liver channel and the *ren mai* channel

The Six Depressions & Transformative Heat

In Chinese medicine, there are six things which may become depressed in the body. These are called the six depressions. They are qi, blood, food, dampness, phlegm, and fire. We have spoken of stagnant qi and static blood above. It is also the qi which moves and transforms food, dampness, and phlegm and all three of these have to do with digestion or spleen/stomach function. Stagnant food is food which is just sitting in the stomach without being transported and transformed. Dampness is liquid which are not be transported and transformed by the spleen, kidneys, and lungs. And phlegm is the by-product of longstanding dampness which eventually congeals. Any of these three yin substances (pathologic or harmful yin, not righteous or good yin) will tend to impede the flow of qi and also clog and weaken the spleen and stomach. Therefore, they can lead to qi stagnation and eventually blood stasis and can impair the spleen's production of blood.

Because qi or life is warm, anything which impedes the flow of qi will tend to cause an accumulation of heat. This heat then warms up the impediment or obstruction transforming it into a Hot accumulation. This is called the theory of similar transformation. It helps explain why so many pathologies are febrile or inflammatory. Qi, blood, food, dampness, and phlegm may all, become, over time, hot stagnant qi, hot static blood, hot food stagnation, damp heat, and hot phlegm. Hot stagnant qi is called transformative or depressive heat.

Because of the close inter-relationships between the various viscera and bowels and qi, blood, and body fluids in Chinese medicine, it is not uncommon to find one or more of these six depressions and transformative heat complicating most chronic disorders. For instance, premenstrual spotting and early periods with dysmenorrhea and clotty, scant discharge suggest liver qi causing blood stasis (pain and clotting) with transformative heat causing both the blood to run recklessly outside its pathway (early menstruation and spotting) and also exhausting or evaporating the blood (scant discharge).

18

Excessive or Abnormal Bleeding

Excessive or abnormal bleeding is an important topic in Chinese medicine. Bleeding is one of six outflows of important substances to which Chinese medicine gives priority in treatment. These six are bleeding, abnormal perspiration, vomiting, diarrhea, excessive urination, and spermatorrhea in men and leukorrhea in women. All these can potentially waste the patient's righteous or healthy energy and nutritive substances. Therefore, Chinese doctors try to check these six outflows as quickly as possible.

According to Chinese medical theory, bleeding can be due to any of four causes. The first and most obvious is traumatic injury. If the vessels or *mai* which channel the blood are severed, the blood will flow out. The second cause of bleeding is based on the reciprocal relationship between the qi and the blood. The qi not only propels the blood but it also holds it within its vessels. Therefore, if qi is vacuous and week, the blood may "fall" or "leak" out of its vessels. The third cause of bleeding is due to heat. Heat may cause the blood to "boil". It then runs recklessly outside its vessels similar to a pot boiling over on a stove. And the fourth cause of bleeding is blood stasis. Although, in some cases where the qi is also relatively weak, blood stasis may just bottle up or "cork" the flow of blood through its vessels. In other cases, where the press of the qi is more insistent, the blood may be forced to flow outside its vessels in an attempt to flow around the stasis or blockage. These four causes of bleeding according to Chinese medical theory are illustrated above in Figure 4 below.

Most women's bleeding associated with endometriosis is due to heat and stagnation. Although, in some women, qi not holding the blood within its vessels may also play a part, especially if the bleeding occurs at the end of or just after menstruation. Menorrhagia, metrorrhagia, hemafaecia, hematuria, epistaxis, and hemoptysis in women with endometriosis are usually diagnosed in traditional Chinese medicine as due either to stagnation, heat, or often a combination of both. We have already seen above how stagnation tends to create heat. Likewise, heat can create stagnation if it exhausts the blood to the point where it no longer has enough volume to maintain its flow. Since the blood volume ebbs and flows cyclically throughout the month, when the blood flow is relatively more full, it may then meet stagnation which was initially

19

created during a period of deficiency or vacuity. This is like a spring torrent meeting a dam of debris deposited on a stream bed when the stream slowed to a trickle during a previous dry spell.

Figure 4: The four causes of bleeding

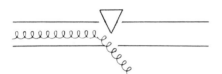

**Bleeding due to traumatic
severance of the vessels**

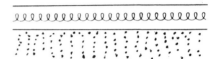

**Bleeding due to qi being
insufficient to hold the blood
within its vessels**

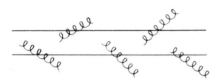

**Bleeding due to heat causing
the blood to run recklessly
outside its vessels**

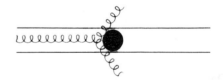

**Bleeding due to stasis forcing
the blood out of bounds or out
of its vessels.**

Chinese Theories about the Percolation of Dampness

The healthy living body is nourished by three humors according to Chinese medicine. These are qi or energy, blood, and liquids. When liquids are correctly metabolized by the lungs, spleen, and kidneys, or rather when they are correctly transported and transformed, to use the Chinese medical terminology, they nourish and lubricate the viscera and bowels and body tissues. However, if body fluids are not transported and transformed properly, they may accumulate and become pathogenic or abnormal dampness.

Dampness is one of the so-called six evils or six pathogens in Chinese medicine. It is turbid and heavy and tends to percolate or seep downwards. Most often, dampness forms because of faulty spleen function in turn due to faulty diet and wrong eating habits, lack of exercise, and excessive worry. Because Dampness is heavy and tends to seep downwards, although it may be produced in the middle burner, the midsection of the body dominated by digestion, it often percolates down into the pelvis. Body fluids are mobilized or transported by the qi. Since the qi moves downward into the pelvis from mid-cycle through menstruation, it is therefore common for this descending qi to aggravate the downward drive of pathogenic dampness into the pelvis premenstrually. If this dampness impedes the flow of qi in the pelvis to the point where the accumulated stagnant qi transforms into heat, this dampness may then become damp heat.

Damp heat in the pelvis premenstrually can cause leukorrhea and vaginal inflammation and itching. However, in women with endometriosis, this downward accumulation of damp heat often manifests as urinary urgency, dysuria, hematuria, polyuria, and nocturia. In some women, it can also manifest as mucous colitis. In this case, if the heat is strong enough, this mucous may also be mixed with blood.

Five Phase Theory

As the lay reader has undoubtedly by now realized, Chinese medical theory is complex. It takes at least four years of study to really understand and internalize all the information and its ramifications presented so far. However, there is still one major Chinese medical theory which needs to be discussed before we can begin to really understand how Chinese medicine diagnoses women with endometriosis. This theory is called in Chinese *wu xing xue*. This is translated as either five element or five phase theory. As it applies to medicine, this theory is mostly used in order to explain certain pathological relationships between the various viscera and bowels. It is also used to prognose the probable evolution of a disease.

According to five phase theory, each of the major viscera is associated with an element or phase. The five phases are wood, fire, earth, metal, and water. These five phases both generate and also check and balance each other, both in the macrocosmic world outside and the microcosmic world internally. Therefore, likewise the viscera both promote or generate each other and also check and inhibit each other according to definite, specific avenues of action.

There are two major avenues of action or cycles of influence according to five phase theory. The first is called the creation or *sheng* cycle. According to this cycle, the liver which is associated with the wood phase is the mother of the heart (fire phase) and the child of the kidneys (water phase). That means the liver receives its nourishment from the kidneys and is responsible for giving sustenance to the heart. Likewise, each of the five major viscera of Chinese medicine is the mother of one viscus and the child of another. These mother-child relationships are diagramed in Figure 5.

The second cycle is called the control or *ke* cycle. It describes how the phases and viscera check each other to maintain homeostasis. According to this cycle, wood, *i.e.*, the liver, controls or checks earth or the spleen. Earth controls water or the kidneys. Water controls fire or the heart. Fire controls metal or the lungs. And metal controls wood or the liver. These control or checking relationships are diagrammed below in Figure 6.

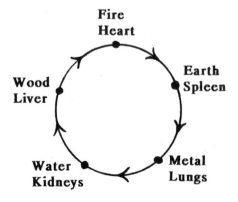

Figure 5: The five phase *sheng* cycle of mother-child relationships

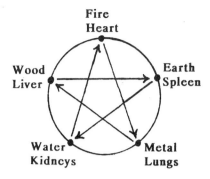

Figure 6: Five phase control (ke) cycle relationships

When we put both the *sheng* and the *ke* cycles together, we have a system of continuous generation with a built in mechanism to stop runaway proliferation. This self-correcting system of generation and control is diagrammed below in Figure 7.

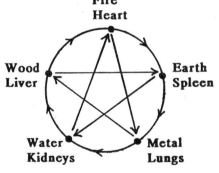

Figure 7: Generation & control cycles operating simultaneously

When this system operates correctly, it maintains the harmonious functioning of all the viscera and bowels of the body. All are promoted but none are allowed to become too strong or out of balance. However, often, due to erroneous diet, lack of exercise, or emotional stress and over-fatigue, some viscera become too strong or replete and others become too weak or vacuous. When this happens, disease will evolve also according to the avenues of action or influence described by the vectors of the *sheng* and *ke* cycles.

In Chinese medicine, one of the statements concerning the liver is that, "*Gan zhu sheng fa*, the liver governs engenderment and effusion." This means that when the liver is functioning normally, it grows flourishingly like a tree in spring. However, it also implies that the liver tends to proliferate effusively. Another Chinese medical dictum reiterates this: "*Mu xi taio da*, wood (the liver) is inclined to spread freely." Not only is the liver inclined to repletion, but it is the temperamental viscus in Chinese medicine. *Gan wei gang zang* means the liver is the "indomitable" viscus. It tends to be indomitable, excess, or replete.

When the liver becomes replete, it may cause manifest symptoms of disease anywhere along the course of its channel or along the course of its paired bowel, the gallbladder's channel. However, it also sets in motion a number of changes in potentially all the other viscera and bowels depending upon such contributing factors as sex, diet, inherent constitutional tendencies, season of the year, phase of the moon, weather, stress, and rest. This explains liver-related menstrual problems including dysmenorrhea, urinary problems, lower abdominal pain and distention, hypochondriac pain and distention, sciatica, flank pain, premenstrual nipple sensitivity, premenstrual irritability, lability, and depression, and premenstrual, one-sided headaches and headaches at the crown of the head.

If the liver "invades" earth along the path of the control cycle, it may cause the stomach to become hot and counterflow and/or the spleen to become weak, deficient, and possibly damp. This can manifest as stomach upset, nausea, and vomiting on the one hand and diarrhea, painful bowel movements, intestinal upset, and constipation on the other. Since typically the liver qi becomes more replete just before the period, before its discharge of blood from the blood chamber (the uterus), this is also when women frequently experience signs and symptoms of the liver's encroachment on the stomach and spleen. See Figure 8.

Long-term spleen vacuity may lead to the accumulation of damp. This, in turn, may lead eventually to diarrhea, dysuria, polyuria, vomiting, leukorrhea, and a heavy sensation in the body in general and especially in the arms and legs. It may also cause headaches which feel like a band of tension surrounding the head. Any or all of these symptoms may become aggravated just

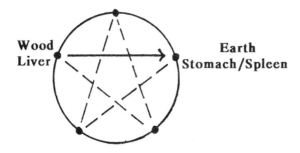

Figure 8. Liver wood invading the spleen/stomach

before the period. Long-term spleen vacuity may also lead to blood vacuity since it is the spleen which initiates the creation of the blood. This may lead to dysmenorrhea, hypomenorrhea, delayed menstruation, amenorrhea, and even infertility. And further, since according to Chinese medicine it is the spleen qi which "lifts" or hold up all the other viscera, long-term spleen qi vacuity may eventually result in prolapse of this so-called central qi. When this happens, the person experiences a bearing-down, dragging pain as if their insides were going to fall out. In terms of menstruation, this is most often experienced towards the end of menstruation when the woman has lost blood and therefore also more qi as well. This pressurey sort of dragging pain is described in *The Merck Manual* as one potential symptom of endometriosis.[29]

Since the spleen is the mother of the lungs, if the spleen is weak, the lungs will also become weak over time. Since the lungs are supposed to control the liver, this weakness allows the liver to flourish or to become even more replete. If the liver gets strong enough and the lungs weak enough, the liver may even "insult" the lungs backwards against the normal flow of the *ke* cycle. This explains perimenstrual hemoptysis according to Chinese medical theory. See Figure 9.

If the liver "catches fire" or becomes so replete as to transform into heat or fire, it will suck up all the yin fuel out of the kidneys, its mother. This leads to yin vacuity of the kidneys. The ultimate yin of the kidneys is the *jing*

---

[29] Ibid., p. 900

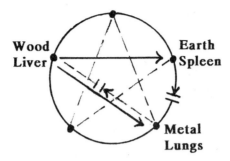

Figure 9. Liver attacks spleen and insults lungs

essence. In Chinese medicine, since some *jing* is required for the creation of new blood, it is said that the *jing* and blood share a common source. This source is the kidney yin. Therefore, kidney yin vacuity can lead to liver blood vacuity causing dysmenorrhea, hypomenorrhea, delayed periods, amenorrhea, and infertility. It can also lead to kidney vacuity polyuria, backache, and menorrhagia. See Figure 10.

And finally, if the liver "burns up", its excessive heat can be transferred to the heart. There it can disturb the *shen* or spirit-consciousness thus causing anxiety, mental agitation, restlessness, fear, and insomnia. Or, through somewhat complex pathways and relationships, it can also cause menorrhagia, metrorrhagia, and hematuria. See Figure 11.

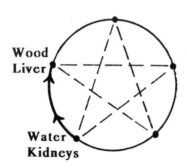

Figure 10. Liver yang exhausting kidney yin according to the *sheng* cycle

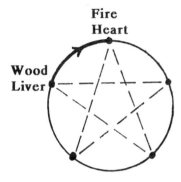

Figure 11. Transmission of liver heat to the heart

The Chinese Diagnosis of Endometriosis

The above heading is a bit misleading since traditional Chinese medicine has no category endometriosis *per se*. However, all the attendant signs and symptoms of endometriosis are traditional disease categories within Chinese medicine. Traditional Chinese gynecology divides disease into four basic categories. These are called *jing, dai, chan, hou* and stand for menstrual diseases, leukorrhea, complaints during pregnancy, and post partum problems. Under menstrual diseases, Chinese medicine does address dysmenorrhea, early, late, and irregular periods, hypo and hypermenorrhea, and perimenstrual bleeding out inappropriate orifices. Infertility is dealt with as a separate, "miscellaneous" gynecological problem. Whereas, dyspareunia or poking pain during intercourse is an important symptom confirming blood stasis. Likewise, diarrhea, vomiting, indigestion, constipation, lower abdominal pain and bloating, hematuria, and dysuria are all disease categories in *nei ke* or Chinese internal medicine.

It is beyond the scope of this book to describe the traditional Chinese differential diagnosis of each and every of the above disease categories or signs and symptoms. Interested readers are referred to *A Handbook of Traditional Chinese Gynecology* for a more complete discussion of the various disease mechanisms of each of these.[30] However, in the Peoples' Republic of China today, there is a move to combine traditional Chinese and modern Western medicines or at least to facilitate their complementing each other. In the PRC, most patients, therefore, receive both a traditional Chinese and a modern Western diagnosis. This is called "dual diagnosis" or diagnosis by both *bian bing*, differentiation of disease, and *bian zheng*, discrimination of pattern of disharmony. Based on this dual diagnosis approach, Dr. Cao Ling-xian and Prof. Tang Ji-fu, both of the Shanghai Gynecology and Obstetrics Hospital, have identified the main, most commonly encountered Chinese disease mechanisms responsible for the development of endometriosis.[31]

Drs. Cao and Tang state that the Western disease endometriosis can be diagnosed as any of four major Chinese *zheng* or patterns of disharmony. Based on my experience of practicing traditional Chinese gynecology for the last ten years, I also agree with this rough division. However, in clinical practice, the professional practitioner must usually discriminate further subdivisions and complications of these basic four patterns. These basic four patterns are: 1) qi stagnation and blood stasis, 2) accumulation of cold causing blood stasis, 3) heat congestion with blood stasis, and 4) qi and blood vacuity with blood stasis.

Qi Stagnation & Blood Stasis

As Dr. Cao Ling-xian says,

> Since Qi is the commander of the Blood and Blood is the mother of the Qi, when Qi circulates, the Blood moves. When Qi stagnates, the Blood stands still.

---

[30] Song Guang-ji & Yu Xiao-zhen, *Zhong Yi Fu Ke Shou Ce (A Handbook of Traditional Chinese Gynecology)*, Fourth Revised Edition, trans. by Zhang Ting-liang and Bob Flaws, Blue Poppy Press, Boulder, CO, 1995

[31] Cao Ling-xian & Tang Ji-fu, "Endometriosis as Treated by Traditional Chinese Medicine", trans. by C.S. Cheung & Carolyn Atkinson, *Journal of the American College of Traditional Chinese Medicine,* S.F., CA, No. 1, 1983, p. 54-57

Endometriosis

Conversely, if Blood stagnates, the Qi also stands still. When the Qi and Blood mutually obstruct in the Extraordinary Vessels, the flow of the Penetrating, Conception, Governing, and Belt Vessels is disrupted (these four being especially important *vis à vis* menstruation and reproduction).[32]

Therefore, qi stagnation leads to blood stasis and blood stasis leads to qi stagnation. And both may lead to pain in the lower abdomen, dysmenorrhea, and infertility. The most common cause of qi stagnation is stress. Stress energetically is qi trying to flow in a certain way or "direction" externally which it cannot freely and patently. This then causes internal congestion of the qi. Since maintaining patency of the qi is primarily the function of the liver, qi stagnation usually results in liver depression. Although stress is the main cause of liver qi (the technical shorthand for liver depression and qi stagnation), stagnant food due to over-eating, blood stasis due to trauma, long-term blood vacuity, and dampness may all impede the free flow of the qi and, therefore, can also contribute to qi stagnation.

This is why the incidence of endometriosis is highest in working women.[33] As Dr. Niels Lauerson states, "Women with endometriosis tend to live stressful lives—this fact cannot be denied."[34] Dr. Lauerson goes on to say that this stress is not just work related but has to do with a number of stressors women experience in contemporary culture.

Beyond job stress, women are juggling the minute-to-minute priorities of work and intimacy, confronting any ambivalence about achievement along with conflicts over dependency on men, figuring out how to achieve a *balance* on a day to day basis—and they are postponing childbirth.[35]

[32] Ibid., p. 54

[33] Lauerson, op.cit., p. 7

[34] Ibid., p. 45

[35] Ibid., p. 7

29

In an article on PMS in *Free and Easy: Traditional Chinese Gynecology for American Women*, I myself have attempted to describe the special stressors in our society creating endemic liver qi in contemporary urban women.

To the idiosyncratic emotional history of the individual must also be added the generalized level of stress and upsetment endemic to our culture. Women's roles are in flux. Old role models have been rejected and new role models may be emotionally unrealistic. Often, modern women feel they should be superwomen. Many women who are single parents or career women try to manifest both traditional female roles of mother and house maker, with the masculine roles of breadwinner and business person. Stress is frustration. It is trying to do too much in a given period of time with inadequate resources. On an energetic level, frustration is an unfluid or impeded flow of qi. Frustration is also an inherently aggressive or angry emotional state of trying to "push the river".

Not only is women's current role in society inherently stressful, but our entire lifestyle generates more stress than I believe the human organism is capable of withstanding without deleterious effect. Background noise from appliances like this electronic typewriter, background music (especially rock n' roll and discordant jazz), television, national and world news, driving in cars, pollution, denatured food, politics, the threat of nuclear war, the breakdown of the family, both nuclear and extended, and the rise of terrifying diseases such as cancer, all cause us more stress than most of us are aware... We have become accustomed to our abnormally high level of ambient stress without having accommodated to it. All this stress adds to any given woman's personal emotional turmoil.[36]

Static blood may be caused by trauma, such as intra-abdominal surgery, blood vacuity, IUDs, abortions, and certain birth control pills in some women. Static blood may also be caused by intercourse during menstruation causing reversed flow of uterine qi and incomplete discharge of menstrual blood. And stagnant blood, as we have seen, can also be due to stagnant qi. The discharge of the period is one way the body seeks to rid itself of stagnant qi and static blood. The blood is mobilized and discharged and if static blood is not too severe, it may be "swept out" with the menstruate. According to Chinese medicine, menstruating and having a baby are essentially analogous energetically. In

---

[36] Flaws, Bob, "Premenstrual Syndrome (PMS)", *Free and Easy, Essays on Traditional Chinese Gynecology for American Women*, Blue Poppy Press, Boulder, CO, 1986, p. 4

both cases, something collects in the uterus and then the body opens to expel or discharge this something, only in the case of pregnancy, this discharge is much greater. Chinese medicine believes that the post partum lochia is, in large part, the body's expulsion of potentially pathogenic qi and blood. Just as the monthly period is a cleansing and release, delivery can also be a cleansing and release but one which is deeper and more profound. Women who postpone childbearing or chose not to have children, therefore, do not experience this cleansing and release. Many doctors used to suggest women get pregnant as a "cure" for endometriosis. When this works, according to Chinese medical theory, it is due to the decongestion of the uterus, vessels, and the liver during the delivery and lochia. The fact that often the endometriosis returns is due to patients' patterns of stress in our society being relatively inescapable.

The signs and symptoms of qi stagnation and liver depression include lower abdominal distention, lower abdominal *crampy* pain, premenstrual breast distention, a stuffy, tight chest, late or irregular periods, and dysmenorrhea at the onset of menstruation which also is crampy rather than stabbing. As the period flows more freely, the cramps disappear. The tongue has a relatively normal coating and may be slightly dark or dusky in color. The pulse is wiry.

The signs and symptoms of blood stasis are stabbing, sharp, fixed, and lancinating pain, clots in the menstrual discharge, the relief of dysmenorrhea after the passing of clots, petechiae or ecchymotic patches on the tongue, prominent blue, varicose, or cyanotic veins on the lower abdomen, possible hemorrhoids or varicose veins on the legs, possible palpable lumps or masses, and poking pain with intercourse. The pulse may be either choppy, irregular, deep, hesitant, or slow.

Some women diagnosed by Western MDs as suffering from endometriosis may only have stagnant qi according to Chinese medicine. But most women with endometriosis have some combination of stagnant q and blood stasis. In such cases, the professional practitioner must assess and diagnose if the qi stagnation is predominant or if the blood stasis is predominant. Also in Chinese medicine, there are several degrees of severity of blood stasis which must be discriminated. Typical complications of qi stagnation and blood stasis endometriosis are blood vacuity and spleen vacuity and/or dampness. When one adds these all together, one may get dysmenorrhea, constipation or

31

diarrhea, sciatica, vomiting, nausea, and indigestion, backache, dyspareunia, scanty, late periods, and symptoms of anemia.

It is important for the lay reader to keep in mind that the diagnosis of qi stagnation and blood stasis endometriosis can only be made on the basis of criteria gathered by the traditional Chinese four examinations. Western medical assessment of the severity of endometriosis through laparoscopy, culdoscopy, ultrasound, and bimanual pelvic examination in no way necessarily corresponds to specific Chinese patterns of disharmony. Chinese medicine does and can only proceed based on a Chinese diagnosis in turn based *solely* on the four *Chinese* methods of diagnosis.

Accumulation of Cold Causing Blood Stasis

Just as cold can congeal water into ice in the outside world, cold can likewise congeal blood into blood stasis internally. In Chinese medicine, qi is life and life is warm. One of qi's five basic functions is to warm the body and its parts. Living qi and cold are mutually opposite. Cold impedes the qi's ability to keep the blood warm and moving. Cold causing blood stasis in the blood chamber (or uterus) or the lower burner (or pelvis) may be due to invasion of cold from without, over-eating cold, raw, and damp foods, or may be due to decline of the person's righteous qi internally with concomitant loss of normal body warmth.

When I was studying with Dr. (Eric) Tao Xi-yu, he said that cold congelation is the most common cause of dysmenorrhea in Chinese medicine. However, in my experience, the incidence of this type of stasis depends upon the geographic locale and upon the lifestyle and nutrition of the patient. In cold, damp climates, cold can invade the lower burner from without. Women working to the point of fatigue in the cold, wet earth with poor or insufficient clothing, no or poor central heating, and a poor diet, as do many female peasants in China, are particularly susceptible to this disease mechanism. Women may especially be invaded by external pathogenic cold during menstruation and during their post partum recuperation when their lower burners have opened for discharge.

Coldness and dampness can also be generated from within by over-eating cold, damp foods. Cold foods include *anything* eaten chilled, frozen, and cold. They also include most raw vegetables and fruits. Damp foods include dairy products, oils, nuts, *sugar*, fatty foods such as pork, and citrus fruits. Therefore, ice cream, chilled milk, and chilled orange juice can all cause chilling and smothering of the fire of digestion. It is the healthy fire of digestion which is the root of the production of day to day qi and therefore warmth. If this fire is chilled by cold foods or doused and·smothered by damp foods, the entire system may become chilled.

Also due to congenital weakness, prolonged illness, extreme fatigue, sexual exhaustion, use of recreational drugs, and due to the natural exhaustion of the aging process, kidney fire can become exhausted or weak. Kidney fire is to spleen warmth what a pilot light is to a stove. Kidney fire is the source of spleen or digestive warmth. Kidney fire is the source of the fire of life of the entire organism. The penetrating, conception, and governing vessels all originate from the uterus anatomically and from the kidneys energetically. If kidney yang or kidney fire declines due to extreme exhaustion, this may cause vacuity cold of the penetrating and conception vessels with attendant blood stasis in the uterus.

The signs and symptoms of accumulation of cold causing blood stasis in the lower burner include cold, fixed pain in the lower abdomen relieved by warmth, a dark, clotty menstrual discharge, aversion to cold, a pale, purplish tongue with a white, wet tongue coating, and a tight, deep, slow, and/or irregular pulse. The period may be late or absent. Lumps or masses may be felt on palpation of the uterus and the patient tends to be chilled. In some cases, they may feel chilled from the waist down as if sitting in cold water. In other cases, the feet may appear blue-purplish in color. If cold and dampness are affecting the spleen, there may be diarrhea, vomiting, loss of appetite, nausea, and leukorrhea. Vacuity cold due to decline of kidney yang may likewise present diarrhea and/or leukorrhea but also typically manifests as low back pain, soreness of the knees, tinnitus, polyuria, and nocturia.

Personally, I do not see much of this type of cold congelation and blood stasis where I practice in Colorado. My patients work indoors, usually have abundant nutrition, live in a dry, temperate to warm climate, are relatively young and in good shape, and therefore tend, if anything, to be hot rather than cold. However, practitioners of Chinese medicine in both the northeast and northwest assure me that they see a significant number of women with menstrual complaints due to cold congelation. When I do see cold congelation and blood stasis in my practice, it is mostly in women who are in their late 30s and 40s. In these cases, spleen qi and kidney yang have both begun to decline and become weak due to aging.

Heat Congestion with Blood Stasis

Most often this Pattern evolves from liver depression qi stagnation. Because qi is warm as part of its inherent description, if it accumulates excessively, it tends to transform into pathologic heat. There are four subdivisions of heat congestion with blood stasis. They are: 1) depressive liver heat and blood stasis, 2) vacuity heat and blood stasis, 3) heat in the stomach and intestines, and 4) mixed hot & cold, replete & vacuity condition.

Depressive liver heat and blood stasis is where long-term liver qi has resulted in blood stasis. At the same time, the liver qi has imploded and transformed into depressive heat. The signs and symptoms of this pattern are the same as for liver qi and blood stasis *plus* signs and symptoms of heat in the liver/-gallbladder. These are bitter taste in the mouth, especially upon arising, irritability and depression, bleeding gums, possible red eyes, dry throat and chronic, recurrent sore throat, possible heartburn, flank pain, scant, darkish, painful urination, a red tongue or tongue rim with a yellowish tongue coating, and a faster than normal, wiry pulse. The periods tend to be early, darkish, rusty, scant, painful, and clotty. There may also be premenstrual and mid-cycle spotting. In addition, there may be yellowish leukorrhea or a thick, white, curdy leukorrhea with vaginal itching and inflammation.

If this heat withers the fluids and yin of the body, the woman will eventually become yin deficiently. At this point, although there are still liver qi and its signs and symptoms, the heat becomes a vacuity heat. That means it becomes like a smoldering fire which continues to burn out of control because everything is so dry. According to Chinese medical theory, yin and yang keep each other in check just as do the qi and blood. When yin becomes weak or consumed, yang tends to flare out of control. Although this heat does not "burn" internally so violently or hotly as does depressive liver heat, it smolders persistently. The signs and symptoms of this type of blood stasis mixed with vacuity heat are, in addition to liver qi signs and symptoms, hot flashes, night sweats, flushing of the cheeks and ears in the late afternoon and early evening, heat in the palms of the hands, soles of the feet, and in the center of the chest, tinnitus, palpitations, possible insomnia, and any other signs and symptoms of liver blood and/or kidney yin vacuity.

The pulse is rapid, fine, and wiry and the left pulse may be generally finer and more evanescent than the right. The tongue is reddish purple, possibly dry, may be cracked, and has a scant, yellow coating. In terms of the menstruation, there may be early menstruation, premenstrual spotting, scant menstruation with clots, delayed menstruation, dysmenorrhea, amenorrhea, and infertility. There is a continuum from depressive liver heat through vacuity heat, therefore, some women may exhibit replete heat symptoms sometimes and vacuity heat symptoms at other times. Careful analysis of the tongue, pulse, and signs and symptoms by a trained professional practitioner, however, should be able to distinguish which is which.

Because the liver and stomach share several close mutual relationships, if the liver becomes replete, the stomach very often gets hot. Heat which builds up in the stomach may also affect the intestines due to their close mutual relationship. Therefore, it is not uncommon to find women with liver qi, blood stasis, and hot stomach and intestines. In such a case, the liver qi and blood stasis signs and symptoms remain relatively the same. In addition, the woman may experience perimenstrual acne, bad breath, mouth sores, constipation, possible hemorrhoids, possible lower abdominal, appendicitis-like pain, and possible hemafecia. the period may be early, voluminous, painful, clotty, and long. In addition, the patient may experience considerable thirst and may be either continuously hungry or have indigestion. Her pulse is rapid and wiry, yet deep in the positions corresponding to the pelvis. The tongue most typically has a thick, yellow fur. This type of stomach heat/liver qi/blood stasis pattern is aggravated by oily, spicy, fried, hot foods and by alcohol.

The last type of depressive heat/static blood scenario associated with endometriosis is a very complicated one. It is where the condition has persisted for a long time and caused various repercussions to a number of different viscera and humors. There is both hot and cold, hot above and cold below or hot inside and cold outside. And there is also repletion and vacuity, repletion static blood but vacuity of either or both qi and blood. Although the sign/-symptom picture is quite variable, the woman may experience intense dysmenorrhea which turns into a dragging pain as the period wears on, vomiting, diarrhea, chills, and cold sweats, but has a red tongue with a yellow coating and a deep, weak, but rapid pulse.

Qi & Blood Vacuity with Blood Stasis

Dr. Cao Ling-xian describes the disease mechanism of this type of endometriosis thus:

> If a patient has Deficiency of Qi, the circulation of Blood will be weak. This, in turn, leads to Blood Stagnation which interferes with the creation of new Blood. This further weakens the Qi and (therefore) the Blood, creating a cycle difficult to break.[37]

There are three main ways of developing this pattern of disharmony here in the United States according to my experience. The first is liver qi causing blood stasis, blood stasis causing blood vacuity, and blood vacuity causing qi vacuity. The second is persistent dampness, worry, and excessive fatigue causing spleen vacuity and dampness thus leading to blood vacuity, blood stasis, and even more qi vacuity. The third is simply overwork, fatigue, and poor nutrition in a woman who is constitutionally already predisposed to qi and blood vacuity. However, no matter what the line of causation, the symptoms tend to be quite similar *vis à vis* the menstruation and menstrual pain.

There is increasing pain as the period progresses ending in a dragging pain in the lower abdomen. The woman may complain of physical and mental fatigue, dizziness, giddiness, lack of appetite, diarrhea, rectal prolapse, hemorrhoids, and tenesmus or bowel cramping. She may desire warmth. Her tongue will typically be pale bluish, swollen, and indented with teeth prints along the sides. Her pulse will be thready, soft, and weak, with maybe a touch of wiry or may also be deep or short. Her period is either early or late, scant or

---

[37] Cao & Tang, op.cit., p. 56

prolonged depending upon which is most vacuous and deficient, qi or blood. The period is also extremely exhausting and the blood may be clotty.

The professional practitioner must further distinguish if qi vacuity is predominant, manifesting as more pronounced fatigue, lethargy, and dragging pain and tenesmus, if blood vacuity is predominant, manifesting as poor memory, palpitations, insomnia, pallor, and scanty, delayed periods, or if vacuity cold of the spleen/stomach is predominant. This manifests as more pronounced diarrhea, lack of appetite, digestive upset, and more pronounced chilling.

Although the laywoman is not expected to be able to keep this plethora of information in her head, nor even to comprehend it thoroughly, it is offered in an attempt to show Western women that Chinese medicine does have a comprehensive and logically systematic description of *all* the various forms and complications of what is diagnosed in modern Western medicine as endometriosis. I feel certain that many women with endometriosis will recognize their own patterns from the above descriptions. And many may be relieved to know that there is a reason, albeit a Chinese reason, for their experiencing what they do.

I would also like to reiterate that all these diagnoses are arrived at by *only* the traditional Chinese four methods of diagnosis: inspection, auscultation/-olfaction, palpation, and questioning. We do not use nor do we need laparoscopies, X-ray exams, culdoscopies, sonograms, biopsies, cystoscopies, thoracentesis, barium enemas, or sigmoidoscopies. Nor do we use or need costly lab exams and analyses. Chinese medicine's diagnostic procedures are non-invasive, non-iatrogenic, low cost, systematic and logical, and also time-tested by one hundred generations of professional practitioners. And, although our diagnostic categories are more general and abstract than modern Western diagnostic categories, they are also more holistic and understandable on the human level of causation. Traditional Chinese diagnoses enlighten and empower us as human beings with human problems. It is relatively easy to translate such a traditional Chinese diagnosis into effective dietary, life-style, and behavior modifications.

The Chinese Prevention & Treatment of Endometriosis

Prevention

Chinese medicine has always traditionally placed great emphasis on prevention. Han Bai-ling, a professor of gynecology in northeastern China, in his *Bai-ling's Gynecology*, gives seven pieces of preventive advice vis a vis menstruation.[38] His first and most important piece of advice is to avoid fear, anger, and excessive emotions in general. Since emotions and qi flow are essentially the same thing, maintaining an even, free flow of moderate emotions is the same as maintaining an even, free flow of qi and blood.

Secondly, Han Bai-ling suggests that just prior to and during menstruation women should not allow themselves to become fatigued. Excessive fatigue means the consumption of the qi and blood and vacuity of the qi and blood during menstruation may injure the penetrating and conception vessels causing blood stasis and thus leading to a number of chronic menstrual diseases.

Third, Dr. Han counsels women not to dwell on their negative thoughts or their frustrations. In particular, it is these thoughts and this stress which causes qi stagnation and leads to blood stasis. The difference between this piece of advice and the first is that excessive emotions of any sort cause erratic qi flow and also tend to transform into heat. Frustration and negativity, on the other hand, lead to stuck qi flow.

Fourth, Dr. Han suggests women to avoid eating cold and raw foods prior to or during their periods. Cold foods depress the digestion thus hindering the production of qi and blood. In addition, Cold constricts the flow of qi and blood. I have treated women for stagnant cold dysmenorrhea caused by eating ice cream the night before the onset of their periods. Raw foods mostly mean salads, raw vegetables, and raw fruits. These tend not only to depress the digestion but also to generate excessive dampness. Prior to the period when

---

[38] Han Bai-ling, *Bai Ling Fu Ke (Bai-ling's Gynecology)*, Heilongjiang, People's Press, Haerbin, PRC, 1983, p. 10

any dampness is percolating down towards the pelvis, excess damp can impede the flow of qi and blood and can then transform into damp heat.

Fifth, Dr. Han suggests that women avoid sex during their periods. This reverses the flow of qi and blood from down and out to up and in and definitely tends to cause the formation of blood stasis. According to Dr. Han, sex during the period damages the penetrating and conception vessels. Han Bai-ling goes on to say that sex during menstruation can lead to uterine bleeding, dysmenorrhea, amenorrhea, and congealed lumps in the pelvis.

Han Bai-ling's sixth piece of advice is for women to avoid strong, vigorous movement or exercise during menstruation so as to prevent qi and blood from leaving their path. Such erratic qi flow may result in menorrhagia, hemoptysis, epistaxis, and uterine bleeding.

Seventh, Han Bai-ling counsels women to eat and drink moderately, to maintain regular waking and sleeping hours, to avoid eating spicy foods, and to try to be happy in order to prevent *all* gynecological problems. In other words, it is Han Bai-ling's opinion that almost all gynecological problems can be prevented *if* a woman maintains mental, emotional, physical, and dietary equilibrium.

Stress Reduction

We, as late twentieth century Westerners, live in a very pressurized, fast-paced, and often frustrating society. Our society does not really support our health. If we are to be healthy, each of us has to take responsibility for ourselves. Based on my ten years of clinical experience, I feel that stress is *the* major cause of most of my patients' problems. Therefore, stress reduction is, I feel, *the* most important part of my patients' preventive and remedial therapy.

There are basically two aspects to stress reduction. The first is life-style modification. This means consciously and deliberately changing whatever external situations we can that are stressing us out. That may mean changing jobs, seeking counseling for relationship problems, changing residence, taking more time off, relinquishing unrealistic goals and expectations, and just in general adopting a slower, more open attitude no matter what we are doing. However, our world is very complex and there are only so many things we can let go of without dropping out of society altogether.

But, besides making necessary changes and adjustments in life situations which are making us sick, we must also teach ourselves consciously and deliberately to relax. Therefore, the second part of stress reduction is deliberate cultivation of the ability to relax through repeated practice. Daily, programmed deep relaxation is, I believe, the single most important element in disease prevention in young and middle-aged, urban and suburban American adults. For deep relaxation to be therapeutically effective, it must fulfill four criteria.

First, it must be done daily. The prescription I give my patients is every day for the first one hundred days without missing a single day. Then, in the next one thousand days, if one misses a few days, that's no big deal. Without routine, day in, day out practice, although each individual session will feel refreshing, there will not be marked progressive and cumulative benefit. Therefore, deep relaxation needs to become a non-discretionary part of every day, as vitally important as eating and sleeping.

Secondly, each day's deep relaxation should last at least twenty, continuous minutes. More than thirty minutes and there is no further health gain for that session. Less than twenty minutes and one will not get any appreciable health result. Therefore, we can say there is a twenty minute threshold to effective, therapeutic deep relaxation.

Third, the deep relaxation should result in complete somatic or physical relaxation and not just mental equipoise. One's whole body, inside and out, should become relaxed, soft, pliable, and at ease. All one's muscles, beginning from the head and working down to the feet, should be allowed to relax, expand, become heavy and warm. Then, in addition, one should calm one's mind through the use of an affirmation, such as the word "relax".

And fourth, having relaxed every muscle in the body, one should center their consciousness in their lower abdomen. One should breathe in and out from their lower abdomen and experience their sense of self from that spot.

If one follows such a regime for one hundred days, their circulation and body temperature will improve, their digestion, elimination, and appetite will improve, and their sleep, mood, and energy will all also improve. Since these are the key criteria for good health in Chinese medicine, one can readily appreciate how important such deep relaxation is in maintaining good health in our hectic world.

Such deep relaxation is not the same as sleep. It is important not to fall asleep until after the twenty minute threshold is reached. After that, it is fine if one chooses to nap for a while or to go to sleep for the evening. Personally, I have found guided deep relaxation tapes, available at most health food and New Age bookstores, to be the easiest and most efficient way of fulfilling this deep relaxation prescription. One simply turns on the tape, lies down, and follows the spoken directions.

After having established the habit of complete and total relaxation, when one is out in the world and problems occur, as soon as one recognizes the tension building in their body, one simply lets go and relaxes. The longer one practices daily deep relaxation, the quicker one is able to let go and clear this tension. According to Chinese medicine, tension is impeded qi and blood and leads to both heat and stagnation. Therefore, the quicker we can let go and relax such tension, the less likely it is that pathologic heat and stagnation accumulate within us.

Aerobic Exercise

Chinese medicine believes that a certain amount of physical exercise is necessary to maintain one's health and to prevent disease. Exercise speeds up a sluggish metabolism and, therefore, increases production of qi and blood. Deficiency of qi and blood can be due just as much to too little exercise as to over-exercise and exhaustion. In addition, regular physical exercise also helps sweep away and disperse any of the six depressions discussed above. Exercise can, as it were, blow out the tubes depressive qi, blood, food, damp, phlegm, and fire. Since these are the main obstructing factors in most chronic, internal disease, one can readily appreciate the healthful and preventive benefits of regular exercise.

As with deep relaxation, I usually write my patients a "prescription" for exercise. For young and middle-aged patients I suggest some sort of aerobic exercise. Any activity which raises the pulse 85% above its resting level and keeps it there for a continuous twenty minutes is aerobic. And, just as with deep relaxation, there is a twenty minute threshold. If one exercises aerobically for from twenty to thirty minutes every other day, one will experience progressively better health. Again, one's circulation and body temperature will improve as will one's digestion, elimination, and appetite. One's mood and energy will improve and so will one's sleep.

In Chinese medicine, we believe that the liver is the primary viscera effected by and involved in stagnant qi. Chinese medicine says the liver stores the blood. When we rest or are physically inactive, the blood returns to the liver from the periphery. When we exercise or are physically active, the qi mobilizes the blood out of the liver. This mobilization helps to sweep away with it any stagnant qi or blood. Also, aerobic exercise benefits the heart and lungs. The lungs, in particular, are said to control the liver according to *ke* cycle energetics. Regular aerobic exercise can keep the lungs strong so that the liver is kept under control. In Chinese medicine, it is the lungs that propel the qi while it is the liver which maintains its free flow and patency. Therefore, it is obvious that the liver and the lungs have a close, reciprocal relationship *vis à vis* the qi. As a specialist in gynecology, patients have consistently reported to me that regular exercise greatly reduces the severity of any symptoms associated with stagnant qi and blood stasis.

Stress, a.k.a. stagnant qi, is like steam in a pressure cooker. We can relieve this pressure by either opening the release valve or turning down the heat. Aerobic exercise is equivalent to opening the release valve within the body. It blows off the steam of accumulated qi due to tension and stress. Deep relaxation is like turning down the heat under the pot. When regular aerobic exercise is coordinated with daily deep relaxation, one has a most effective and efficient combination for preventing stress-induced disease. The key to both is regularity and perseverance. Deep relaxation should be done every day and aerobic exercise every other day or not less than every seventy-two hours.

Diet

Chinese medicine places great importance on diet. We manufacture qi and blood to power and nourish us from a combination of three basic sources. The air we breathe is mixed or "combusted" with the food and liquids we eat and drink catalyzed by our innate constitutional or inherent energy. There is little we can do about the air we breathe and breathing is best left as an unconscious activity. Likewise, our constitutional or inherent energy is what it is and is not subject to much conscious modification by us. But what we eat, how much we eat, and how we eat are all within our control and can greatly affect our health and well-being.

To understand Chinese dietary theory, one must understand the Chinese concept of digestion. Everything that is eaten and drunk is first received by the stomach. The stomach is likened to a pot on a stove. Its job is to cook the digestate similar to a sour mash. As the digestate is "cooked" by the stomach, it is "rottened and ripened". The finest essence of the digestate is then distilled by the spleen and sent up to the lungs and heart to be transformed into qi and blood respectively. Therefore, before any nutritive essence can be absorbed by the body, the food eaten must be turned into 100° degree soup in the stomach.

This explains Chinese medicine's emphasis on cooked as opposed to raw foods. Cooking is predigesting. By cooking, we begin on the outside of the body the process of rottening and ripening the stomach must continue on the inside. Cooking makes the nutrients in foods more easily assimilable. Since the process of digestion is characterized as a process of warm transformation, eating cooked, warm foods results in a greater net gain. As the pure arises to be transformed into qi and blood, the turbid residue of the digestate is descended to be eventually excreted from the body. If the pure and turbid do not separate completely and efficiently, dampness, phlegm, and stagnant Food are created which obstruct the flow of qi and the creation of blood and generally gum up the works.

Likewise, since life is qi and qi is warm, most food we eat should not only be warm in temperature but also warm in nature. Chinese medicine identifies the inherent temperature of each food's qi. Food can either be hot, warm, neutral, cool, or cold. Mostly our diet should be composed of warm and neutral foods. And naturally, most foods are warm or neutral in temperature. However, many fruits and some vegetables, such as cucumbers, celery, and lettuce, are cool or cold. For a description of the temperatures of one hundred fifty commonly eaten foods, the interested reader is referred to my and Honora Lee Wolfe's *Prince Wen Hui's Cook: Chinese Dietary Therapy*.[39]

In addition, drinking too much liquid and especially cold liquids with meals dilutes the soup and smothers the fire of digestion. A teacup of warm, boiled water, tea, or broth aids digestion, but an eight ounce glass of iced water or soda puts the fire of digestion out temporarily. Therefore, in Asia it is traditionally believed that for optimal digestion the stomach should be half full of food, one quarter full of liquid, and one quarter empty to allow for proper churning of the digestate.

There are also certain specific foods which should be eaten in great moderation by everyone and especially by women prone to endometriosis. Sugar is extremely sweet. The sweet flavor, according to Chinese medicine, goes right to the spleen and also promotes the secretion of body fluids. Sugar is so sweet that it "blows out" the spleen. Rather than supplementing or strengthening the spleen as does the natural, low concentrated sweet flavor of most grains, meats, and vegetables, concentrated sweet weakens the spleen and therefore the healthy creation of qi and blood. In addition, sugar and other concentrated sweets such as honey, molasses, maple syrup, and various malt syrups, also tend to create dampness due to over-secretion of body fluids. This dampness then hinders the spleen function even more. The *Nei Jing*, the oldest classic of Chinese medicine, says that the sweet flavor helps to relax the liver and so it is natural for people with liver depression and qi stagnation to crave the sweet flavor. Unfortunately, when this craving is indulged by eating something so extremely sweet as sugar, although it may give temporary respite, it only makes the entire situation that much more complicated and difficult to remedy.

---

[39] Flaws, Bob & Wolfe, Honora Lee, *Prince Wen Hui's Cook, Chinese Dietary Therapy*, Paradigm Publications, Brookline, MA, 1983

Other foods that can create dampness are nuts, oils, and fats, chocolate, beef and pork, dairy products, eggs, and citrus fruits, pineapples, apples, and pears. Women whose spleens are chronically damp due to long-term spleen vacuity in turn aggravated by liver qi should be very careful not to over-eat damp-producing foods. Alcohol is also dampening. It is also hot. Therefore, it tends to create not only dampness but damp heat.

Most spices are hot in nature or, at best, warm. In small amounts they, therefore, aid digestion, but, if over-eaten, they tend to create replete heat in the stomach and liver. Most Western women with endometriosis or any disorder with a component of liver qi must be careful of hot, spicy foods. Spices and pungent foods do decongest stagnant qi temporarily, but they also tend to waste the blood and over-heat a typically over-heated system. Alcohol likewise temporarily disperses stagnant qi, but it too aggravates any pathologic heat.

One other food which is a disaster for women with any Chinese liver condition is coffee. This includes both caffeinated coffee and de-caff. Coffee disperses stagnant qi but wastes the blood and yin. As a qi decongestant, it is extremely effective short-term as is alcohol to an alcoholic. Coffee gives a sense of energy and get up and go by freeing up stuck qi. But in the process, it also liberates stored *jing* or essence in the kidneys and, therefore, is deleterious to the health over-all. Although I personally do not see *any* good, healthy reason for drinking coffee, women who experience any kind of menstrual, reproductive tract, or breast disorders should avoid coffee at all costs. Although caffeinated coffee has an even worse effect than de-caff, it is not the caffeine alone that is the offending substance. There are many volatile oils in the coffee bean which as a whole cause the problem. Relatively speaking, green tea has caffeine but does not cause the same problems as even de-caffeinated coffee. In fact, green tea has many positive health benefits. Coffee, like sugar and alcohol is an addictive substance and is not easy to relinquish. Placing a drop of White Flower Oil on the tip of the tongue when the coffee craving strikes can help alleviate this dependency.

This all means that women living in a temperate climate should eat mostly cooked grains and vegetables. They should probably eat small amounts of meat, once every other day or so. By small amounts, I mean not more than two ounces per serving. Also, meat broths are very nutritious without the heaviness and dampness of eating the flesh itself. Soups are very healthy since they already are extremely digestible. One can also eat occasional fruits, some nuts, and some dairy if one's digestion and elimination are sound and if they are not prone to phlegm and dampness. This is similar to the Pritikin diet or the Macrobiotic diet except without the emphasis on exotic "Japanese" foods often encountered in the latter. This is the diet most humans have eaten in temperate climates for thousands, if not tens of thousands of years. When looked at through the lens of history, our modern American diet is a recent fad of not much more than fifty years duration. By returning our emphasis to cooked grains and cooked, fresh vegetables, we fuel ourselves on the diet our bodies evolved on.

This is also basically the diet recommended in the National Research Council's *Diet and Health: Implications for Reducing Chronic Disease Risk.* According to this recently released, 1,300 page document, fats should make up no more than 30% of the total day's calories and saturated fats should only make up a third of that. Complex carbohydrates which are found in vegetables, legumes, and grains should make up at least 55% of daily calories. Protein for adults should *not* exceed any more than twice the daily recommended allowance (0.8 grams per kilogram of ideal body weight). Also according to this report, alcohol should be limited to one ounce per day and salt to a maximum of approximately one teaspoon per day.[40] Chinese medicine has been counseling such moderation in diet for well over a thousand years.

These three therapies described above—deep relaxation, aerobic exercise, and dietary therapy—are the three cornerstones of both preventing the arisal of disease and of treating chronic disease. Sun Si-miao, the most famous Chinese physician of the Tang dynasty (circa 700 CE), said that disease should first be treated by diet and lifestyle modification. If that does not cure the problem, only then should acupuncture and herbal medicine be employed. Sun Si-miao was writing in a simpler time and modern patients both want and probably

---

[40] *Time Magazine*, NYC, March 13, 1989, p. 51-52

need more professional intervention at the same time as they change their diet and lifestyle. Still, Sun's advice concerning the primary importance of these three, free therapies remains true to this day. Lucy Mall, writing in *Vegetarian Times*, states:

Conventional medicine has ignored prevention until very recently, and the results are clear. Chronic illness is now responsible for more than 80 percent of all deaths and an even higher percentage of all total disability, states Robert A. Anderson, M.D., in *Wellness Medicine*. Many studies confirm that lifestyle factors, which are largely preventable, are the cause of debilitating disorders. In a Massachusetts study, for example, four risk factors for chronic disease—lack of exercise, smoking, overweight, and alcohol use—may account for over half the annual deaths in the United States, the authors concluded.[41]

In my experience, as much as 75% of all overt symptomology can be relieved in the majority of cases after three months of the above three, self-administered therapies. It is very common for me to meet patients on the street whom I have not seen for some time. Often they tell me that when their signs and symptoms flare up or return, all they have to do is get these three free therapies back on line again and soon their condition returns to normal. Sometimes they tell me this almost apologetically, as if my feelings will be hurt because they do not need my professional assistance. However, just the contrary, this is what causes me the greatest delight. The same Sun Si-miao also said the Superior Physician does not just treat disease but teaches society and helps form the intentions of humanity.

These three free therapies—deep relaxation, aerobic exercise, and dietary modification and moderation—are the keys to preventing dysmenorrhea and endometriosis. They are also the first and most important parts to the treatment of these conditions by full-spectrum, holistic, Chinese medicine. If women with dysmenorrhea, endometriosis, and infertility adjust their diets and lifestyles according to the above guidelines, then Chinese herbal medicine and acupuncture can bring the benefits of Chinese medicine into full display.

---

[41] Moll, Lucy, "Playing God, When Medicine Plays Monopoly", originally printed in *Vegetarian Times, Nexus*, Boulder, CO, No. 30, Spring, 1989, p. 42

Avoiding Iatrogenesis

Iatrogenesis means the causation of disease by faulty or incorrect treatment. Unfortunately, all too often in the West, iatrogenesis plays a part in the development of endometriosis and infertility. Rarely, however, is this due to negligence or incompetence on the part of Western physicians. Rather, it is due to the short-sighted, incomplete view of modern Western medicine. By focusing too narrowly and mechanically on the minutiae of matter, Western medicine fails to see the bigger picture and therefore often its interventions, although seemingly brilliant short-term, turn out to cause complications as time goes by.

When discussing blood stasis above, I mentioned that IUDs, pelvic surgery, abortions, and some birth control pills in some women can lead to the formation of blood stasis. This opinion is based on analyzing, according to the theories and diagnostic parameters of traditional Chinese medicine, the signs and symptoms of a large number of female patients which have arisen after such procedures. All too often, signs of blood stasis which were absent before such procedures or treatments manifest after them. This is especially so in women who already suffer from either liver depression and qi stagnation or vacuity of the blood. Therefore, whenever possible, it is best to avoid these quick fixes. In the case of lower abdominal surgery, sometimes this is necessary in order to save a life in an emergency situation. However, if traditional Chinese medicine is resorted to at an early stage, most intra-abdominal surgery can be avoided. For instance, I treat approximately two cases of intestinal abscess, what Western medicine calls appendicitis, per year with Chinese medicine, acupuncture and herbs, and none of my patients in ten years have required an appendectomy. IUDs, birth control pills, discretionary surgery, such as tubal ligation, and abortions are all matters of choice, not necessity. Condoms, diaphragms, and spermicidal jellies and foams have far fewer iatrogenic consequences than IUDs, abortions, tubal ligations, and birth control pills.

In addition, the Western medical treatment of most pelvic inflammations is incomplete and can lead to chronic sequelae. Most pelvic inflammations, such as salpingitis (PID), bladder and vaginal infections, and venereal diseases, are treated by Western medicine with antibiotics. Antibiotics are, for the most part, extremely cold medicines. Since most pelvic infections and inflammations are hot diseases, at least in part, these cold medicines can counteract and neutralize this pathogenic heat. However, according to Chinese medicine, not all pelvic infections are due to heat or are hot in nature and those that are may also have other energetic components. For instance, some women who are diagnosed as suffering from PID by Western medicine are diagnosed as having prolapse of central qi and vacuity and stasis of blood by Chinese medicine. Prolapse of central qi means spleen qi vacuity and since most antibiotics weaken the spleen qi, as evidenced by their tendency to cause diarrhea or loose stools, this treatment only aggravates such conditions. Likewise, many pelvic infections are not only hot but also damp and may be additionally complicated by stagnant qi and blood stasis. Antibiotics may get rid of the heat but do not address the dampness nor the stagnation. Since, in Chinese medicine, dampness can cause heat, such infections can become chronic and recurrent. In addition, since chronic stagnation and dampness both impede the production of fresh blood and qi, this scenario can eventually become complicated by qi and blood vacuity as well, for which antibiotics only make the long-term situation more and more recalcitrant.

The importance of such iatrogenesis due to sort-sighted and incomplete Western medical treatment should not be over-looked. Dr. Richard L. Sweet, writing on pelvic infections and infertility in *Progress in Infertility*, states:

> The United States is in the midst of an epidemic of sexually transmitted diseases. Between 1950 and 1975, the incidence of reported gonorrhea in the total United States population tripled to its hyperendemic rate of more than a million cases reported annually. Because of under-reporting, it is estimated that over three million cases occur each year in the United States. In addition, chlamydiae have become recognized as causing an even more commonly sexually transmitted disease, and recent estimates suggest that 3 to 5 million cases of chlamydial infection occur annually in this country. As a result of this epidemic and the widespread use of the intrauterine contraceptive device, the incidence of acute salpingitis has also increased. Acute salpingitis is the most prevalent important complication of sexually transmitted pathogens. An estimated 1 million women a year are treated for it in the United States. Approximately 250,000 women are

hospitalized each year with the primary and secondary diagnosis of salpingitis or pelvic inflammatory disease (PID)... One fourth of all women who have had acute salpingitis will experience one or more long-term sequelae. The most common and most important is involuntary infertility which occurs in about 20 percent.[42]

It is interesting to note that many women with endometriosis have been previously diagnosed and treated for PID. These two are different Western diseases but are often diagnosed as one and the same pattern of disharmony in Chinese medicine. The good news is that Chinese medicine does treat holistically and comprehensively most vaginal, bladder, pelvic, and cervical inflammations and infections through a combination of herbal medicine and acupuncture. When Chinese medicine does treat these conditions, it treats the entire woman or the complete condition. It does not just clear heat but also, if necessary, eliminates dampness, destagnates the qi and blood, and supplements any energy or organs which have become weak or vacuous. Therefore early treatment of acute pelvic and urogenital infections by a comprehensive and holistic medicine is important for preventing more serious, recalcitrant disorders, including infertility. Readers interested in a further discussion PID and Chinese medicine are referred to my *Free and Easy, Traditional Chinese Gynecology for American Women*.[43]

Some, if not most women reading this section will undoubtedly have used in their past some of the Western treatments discussed above. However, they should not be depressed by this. Although such choices and treatments may have contributed to their present situation, these choices and treatments are in the past. What's done is done. Happily, Chinese medicine can treat and reverse most of the sequelae of such short-sighted treatments.

I also do not mean to give the impression that all Western medicine is iatrogenic or bad. It is not. When its interventions are truly appropriate and called for, they are quick and extremely effective. The problem is that the heroic measures of Western medicine are too often resorted to too soon. One

---

[42] *Progress in Infertility*, Third Edition, S.J. Behrman, Robert W. Kistner, & Grant W. Patton, eds., Little, Brown & Co., Boston, 1988, p. 25

[43] Flaws, *Free and Easy*, op.cit.

should first use more natural and organic methods of treatment when the problem is in its formative stages. Only when such gentler therapies have failed or when the situation is critical should the "heavy guns" of the Western medical armamentarium be brought into play.

Remedial Treatment

Chinese Herbal Medicine

Chinese medicine's main professional therapy is internally administered herbal medicine. Actually, herbal medicine is a bit of a misnomer. Although most of the 5,000 medicinal substances in Chinese medicine come from various plants, Chinese medicine does also use both naturally occurring mineral substances and animal by-products. All these ingredients are seldom used singly. Most often they are combined into formulas comprised of from eight to fifteen ingredients. In such a formula, the ingredients work synergistically. Some of the ingredients boost each other's beneficial, therapeutic effect. Other ingredients are meant to negate possible side-effects. And yet other ingredients insure that the right effect is obtained in the right part of the body.

The most common traditional method of administration is as a decoction. This means the herbs are boiled in water for forty-five minutes to an hour or more. After straining off the liquid, this "tea" is drunk several times per day. Other methods of administration include pills, powders, liquid and dried extracts, and syrups. Which method of administration is used will depend on the individual patient's diagnosis and case. However, commonly, one begins treatment with strong decoctions. As their symptoms improve and progress is made, they are then moved to powders, pills, or extracts for easier, long-term administration.

The practitioner of traditional Chinese medicine composes a customized herbal prescription specifically for the individual patient. He or she begins with the diagnosis of the disease category and the individual patient's pattern of disharmony. He or she then modifies the formula for the patient's idiosyncratic signs and symptoms and individual constitution. Therefore, a dozen women all with a Western diagnosis of endometriosis may each receive a different herbal formula. In addition, this formula is adjusted approximately once per week based on where the woman is in her menstrual cycle, what symptoms are currently manifesting, the season of the year, the phase of the moon, the weather, and any of a number of other individualized considerations.

When prescribed correctly based on an individualized Chinese energetic diagnosis, Chinese herbal medicine is free from *any* side-effects. Since Chinese medicine sees the organism as a whole, throwing one part of the body out of balance in an attempt to heal another part makes little sense. Chinese doctors are constantly up-dating and modifying their patients' treatment since the patient is constantly changing in relationship to their environment.

Therefore, it is very important for the patient to keep their Chinese physician constantly informed about all their body functions and symptomatic experiences. Likewise, it is also important that the Chinese doctor monitor their patients' pulse and tongue on a regular basis since an accurate traditional Chinese medical diagnosis primarily depends upon the comparison of a patient's signs and symptoms, tongue, and pulse.

In my experience, women with endometriosis generally require from three to six months of intensive Chinese herbal therapy to achieve substantial amelioration in their condition. In cases where stagnation is the more prominent issue, herbal therapy is "heaviest" from mid-cycle through the onset of the period. During the post menstruum the woman may not have to take any Chinese herbal medication. In cases where vacuity of the qi and blood is more prominent, herbal therapy is typically heaviest during and just after the period. Women whose condition is mostly just replete, as in stagnant qi and blood stasis, usually get better as a straight progression. Each period is better than the one before. Women whose condition begins as vacuity, however, may seemingly get worse as they are getting better. As the vacuity is supplemented, this bigger volume of qi and blood may encounter an underlying tendency to stagnation of the qi. In this case, the symptoms of vacuity, such as dragging pain and fatigue, improve but are replaced by stronger dysmenor-rhea at the onset of menstruation. This, in fact, is a good sign and shows substantial improvement in the over-all condition. It also indicates that there is still work to be done.

Some women may at first think that Chinese herbal medicine is expensive. It can cost, depending upon the method of administration, dose, and prescrip-tion, from one to four or even five dollars per day. However, when compared to the cost of most Western drugs and medical procedures, the net cost of Chinese medicine is relatively cheap. Why some Western women may hesitate or balk at spending this much money on Chinese herbs is that they feel Chinese medicine is just an experiment. Since they are not sure it will work for them, it seems an expensive risk. However, I can say conclusively that Chinese medicine is *not* experimental when it comes to treating gynecological problems, that it does work when practiced and administered properly, and that, in the long run, it definitely is cheaper and more effective than Western medicine.

Some women may also find the taste of Chinese herbal decoctions very bitter and unpleasant. In China there is a saying, the bitterer the brew, the better the medicine. However, that may be small consolation for the modern Western patient. But, I can say based on my own and my patients' experience, when a Chinese herbal prescription matches exactly an individual patient's condition, after the first few doses, the body recognizes the benefit of the decoction and even comes to crave the taste of such bitter brews. When this happens, it is a very encouraging sign. Then, if and when the same formula begins to taste bad again, it is a sign that the current prescription is no longer exactly right and needs to be modified or changed completely to a different formula.

Chinese herbal medicine is a fine art which takes a great deal of education and years of practice to master. Chinese herbal ingredients are medicinals. They are medicine and are not just inconsequential dietary supplements. As such, they must be prescribed by professional practitioners specifically trained in Chinese herbalism and their prescription must be based on traditional Chinese theories and a traditional Chinese energetic diagnosis. Chinese doctors have developed and refined this system over two thousand years. When Westerners attempt to use Chinese medicinals on the basis of a Western diagnosis or Western medical theories alone, either the treatment is not successful or, in fact, iatrogenic complications are caused. Chinese medicine may be "herbal", but it is strong medicine nonetheless. When practiced and prescribed professionally and correctly, it is strongly beneficial.

Acupuncture

Acupuncture is the other main, professionally administered therapy of traditional Chinese medicine. Acupuncture is the insertion of extremely fine needles into specific locations on the body called acupoints. According to Chinese medical theory, qi and blood flow through the body over discrete channels and vessels. These *jing mai* are relatively the same for everyone regardless of race. Located on these pathways are points or "switches" at which the energy traveling through them can be manipulated and therapeutically adjusted. Inserting needles into these points is similar to flicking switches or circuit breakers in an electrical system. The acupuncturist can either send more or less energy to an organ or area of the body, can direct the qi, blood, and body fluids, can speed up or slow down these humors, and can warm them up or cool them down.

The needles are inserted from just barely under the skin to a half inch, one inch, or even more in depth. Patients may experience the slightest pinch on insertion and then any of several sensations as the needle touches the point which is below the skin. These sensations can include tingling, heat, distention, heaviness, soreness, or an electrical, nervy feeling. These are all good signs that the needle has "tapped the qi" and that something therapeutic is happening. Usually somewhere around eight points are needled in a single treatment (often bilaterally) and the needles may be left in place for from fifteen to twenty minutes as the patient lies on the table. If the acupoints have been correctly selected, typically patients will begin to breathe very deeply. They will relax deeply and may even fall asleep. These are all good signs the treatment is restoring balance to the body and is freeing stuck and stagnated energy and tension.

In my experience in treating women with endometriosis, I find that acupuncture is most effective when administered every other day for three to four treatments during the premenstruum or from whenever marked premenstrual signs and symptoms appear. When acupuncture is combined with internally administered Chinese herbal medicine, it is usually only necessary for the first three months of treatment. By that time, so much improvement has been achieved that acupuncture is usually no longer necessary. However, if the patient is coming in regularly for consultation for herbal modifications, acupuncture may then be given once per week or so to aid in general balancing.

Dr. Kathyrn Schroetenboer, in *Freedom From Menstrual Cramps*, dismisses acupuncture as quackery.[44] However, a federal district court judge in Texas has ruled that acupuncture is no more experimental than the Chinese language. In fact, acupuncture is extremely effective in treating dysmenorrhea. In a study done by Dr. Joseph M. Helmes in Berkeley, traditional Chinese acupuncture achieved a 90.9% rate of success in treating dysmenorrhea.[45] I have often treated with acupuncture women carried into my office or lying in heaps on their floors at home incapacitated and almost insensible with severe dysmenorrhea. In every single instance, their cramps were relieved entirely or markedly diminished to tolerable levels within fifteen to twenty minutes after insertion of the needles.

In general, the more stagnant qi and blood stasis are part of a woman's diagnosis, the more useful acupuncture is in an over-all Chinese medical treatment plan. When cold congelation or vacuity cold are more prominent in a woman's Chinese diagnosis, moxibustion may be done instead of or in

---

[44] Schroetenboer, Kathryn & Subak-Sharpe, Genell J., *Freedom from Menstrual cramps*, Pocket Books, NYC., 1981, p. 58-59

[45] Lauerson, op.cit., p. 106

combination with acupuncture. Moxibustion is the warming of acupoints with a burning punk or "cigar" made of Herba Artemisiae Argyii. This herb is particularly effective in warming cold and also in supplementing the qi which is itself inherently warm. The burning punk is held an inch or so over the acupoint until a deep, penetrating heat is felt. The acupoint itself should become warm to the touch and quite red. However, the skin should not be scorched nor should any blister be raised in usual practice. Sometimes patients are even instructed how to apply such moxibustion on their own at home, thus increasing the total number of treatments without increasing the number of office visits and therefore cost.

Here in the West, most practitioners of traditional Chinese medicine are also trained acupuncturists. There is a National Commission for the Certification of Acupuncturists in the United States which offers a national board certification exam. Acupuncturists who are nationally board certified typically append Dipl.Ac. for Diplomate of Acupuncture after their names. Just as one would not hire a plumber to do electrical wiring, patients should best receive acupuncture from trained, credentialed, professional acupuncturists. Also, because of the advent of AIDS, most Western acupuncturists use ethylene oxide gas sterilized, disposable needles. This virtually eliminates *any* possibility of cross infection through contaminated needles. In addition, more and more insurance companies are willing to reimburse for acupuncture since it is such a cost-effective therapy.

Vitamins & Supplements

Potentially any substance which can be described according to the categories and rubric of Chinese medicine can be logically incorporated into a traditional Chinese treatment plan. A substance does not have to have originated in China for it to be an acceptable part of Chinese medicine. In fact, many "Chinese" herbal ingredients were or are still imported from foreign countries, for instance American Ginseng. If a substance can be understood as if it were a Chinese herb, then it can be added to the traditional Chinese pharmacopeia. Vitamins and minerals are a case in point.

Women suffering from endometriosis often benefit from adding B vitamins, C and bioflavanoids, and mineral supplements to their daily regime. B vitamins supplement yin and blood, calm the spirit, and relax the liver. Vitamin C regulates the qi and also clears heat. And minerals, such as calcium and selenium, calm the spirit and settle anxiety and restlessness. Knowing this, they can be just as logically incorporated into a Chinese treatment plan as Ginger, Mint, Licorice, Bupleurum, or Dang Gui.

Since vitamin and mineral metabolism is synergistic, I recommend taking a well-balanced multivitamin, multimineral supplement with a strong dose of Bs. In general, I do not suggest megadoses of vitamins and minerals since it is very easy to inadvertently upset the delicate vitamin metabolism. In particular, since many Western women have some degree of spleen vacuity and since vitamin C can weaken the spleen and cause diarrhea if taken in too large a dose, it should not be taken in such large doses that it makes the stools too loose. Since the endemic stress within our modern society is, I believe, beyond the healthy carrying capacity of most individuals and because of pervasive air, water, and soil pollution, I do think taking some vitamin and mineral supplements are appropriate and that this in no way violates the internal logic or consistency of traditional Chinese medicine. Already, some Western practitioners of Chinese medicine are incorporating vitamins, minerals, and amino acids into traditional Chinese herbal formulas and with good results.

Oriental Aroma Therapy

Although professional Chinese medicine emphasizes internally administered herbal medicines and acupuncture, it has available to it a full range of healing modalities, one of which is aroma therapy. This is the inhalation of various smokes and steams. Aroma therapy has fallen somewhat out of use in China itself but has been kept alive in Tibet. Personally, I find aroma therapy using a Tibetan-made herbal incense of definite benefit in alleviating the mental and emotional symptoms attendant to liver depression and qi stagnation.

Persons suffering from liver qi are often depressed and often irritable. Their emotions come in fits and starts as the qi first backs up behind the congestion and then vents when it accumulates sufficient pressure. Therefore, people with liver qi are by turns both irritable and morose. Instead of their emotions being very stable, their emotions fluctuate greatly and therefore can be described as being very labile.

Although Western practitioners of Chinese medicine usually translate the word qi as energy as a way of simplifying this profound concept for their Western patients, qi means more than just energy. It also carries the connotations of wind and spirit as well, in the Greek sense of *pneuma* and the Latin *spiritus*. Therefore, qi is closely related to both aromas and breathing. We are all familiar with how potent a fragrance can be in eliciting a memory pregnant with emotion. Emotion is just the subjective experience of qi. Also, most of us have felt how our breathing becomes fast and shallow when we become upset or uptight. Because of the close connection of the qi to breathing, it is not surprising that in the Orient medicinal incenses have been formulated to specifically treat emotional disequilibrium.

In Chinese and Tibetan medicines, Lignum Aquilariae Agallachae (*Chen Xiang*) is a medicinal ingredient which regulates the qi. It is an extremely aromatic and precious wood which is often too expensive to use in internally administered decoctions (at least its higher quality grades). However, in incense only a very small amount of this wood is necessary in order to produce a definite psychological effect. Lignum Aquilariae is one of the main ingredients in a Tibetan medicinal incense formula known as Agar 31. This incense is manufactured for American distribution under the name Nirvana Incense and is available in many health food and New Age bookstores, especially those specializing in Tibetan Buddhist books.

Women experiencing pronounced PMS emotional hypersensitivity, depression, irritability, and insomnia can light a small piece of this incense and inhale its smoke for approximately ten minutes. This can take the edge off these emotional symptoms and discomfort due to erratic and congested qi flow. Since many women with endometriosis and infertility suffer from periodic bouts of emotional lability, such aroma therapy is a useful adjunctive therapy. If Nirvana Incense is not locally available, simply burning a small piece of Lignum Aquilariae on an incense charcoal can also offer relief. All Chinese herb stores carry this ingredient and most Western practitioners of Chinese medicine who have their own dispensaries will be able to furnish their patients with this ingredient.

Combining Chinese & Western Remedial Therapies

Modern Western medicine is the currently dominant medicine in developed nations. Most Western patients come to practitioners of Chinese medicine with an already established Western medical diagnosis. Many patients are also currently taking allopathic medicines based on their Western medical diagnosis. Therefore, the question often arises whether or not to continue this allopathic medication or treatment while at the same time engaging in Chinese medicine.

This is a complex question and its answer depends upon a number of individual factors. Essentially, however, if the Western medicine is free of side-effects and seems to be working, then it can be continued along with Chinese medical treatment if the patient so desires. If the Western medicine or treatment is causing side-effects, then either of two approaches can be taken. Either Chinese medicine can be administered to mitigate and treat these side-effects or the Western medicine should be discontinued and Chinese medicine relied on alone.

If a Western medicine or treatment can be understood in Chinese medical terms and according to Chinese medical theory, then the Chinese-style practitioner can analyze the usefulness and the appropriateness of the Western treatment as if it were any other therapy within Chinese medicine. Chinese medicine originated in China but it is a universally valid theory and medical system and potentially any medicinal substance or therapy may be added to its panoply of modalities. For instance, although Chinese herbal medicine and acupuncture can, in theory, reduce masses and resolve tumors, it often does so slowly or poorly. In such cases, it may often be wiser to have such masses or tumors surgically excised quickly and efficiently and then use Chinese medicine to speed recuperation and to rectify the underlying energetic process which gave rise to the mass in the first place. Since this process is not aborted by surgery, it still needs to be dealt with lest this same process give rise to the formation of another neoplasm somewhere else. It has been estimated that the recurrence rate for endometriosis after conservative surgery (not a hysterectomy) to be as high as 40%. After radical hysterectomy, the rate of recurrence may even reach 97%.[46]

Many Western drugs have simply too many side-effects for Chinese medicine to consider them a wise and humane therapy. Modern Western doctors often consider certain side-effects to be acceptable, harmless, and inconsequential. Chinese medicine does not. Any aberration to the over-all functioning of the organism over time may have serious and even disastrous consequences. This is based on Chinese medicine's thoroughgoing holism in which every part and function of the body is interconnected. When a Western drug causes side-effects which Chinese medicine considers debilitating and counterproductive and when Chinese medicine alone can reasonably be expected to treat the original problem without side-effects, then I suggest using traditional Chinese medicine alone and discontinuing the Western medication.

In the 365 women study initiated by the Endometriosis Association of Milwaukee, all the women were treated with Danazol, an androgen which creates pseudomenopause and which is the current allopathic treatment of first choice for endometriosis. Of these 365 women, *all of them* reported side-effects.[47] The side-effects of Danazol include hot flashes and flushing, acne, growth and darkening of facial hair, masculinization of voice, liver dysfunction, edema, enlargement of the clitoris, vaginitis, vulvitis, weight gain,

---

[46] Older, op.cit., p. 107

[47] Ibid., p. 185

muscle cramps, and decreased breast size. Some of these side-effects may be, according to Western medicine, irreversible.

The disease mechanism theory of Chinese medicine can explain why each of these side-effects arise in a given woman and which women are likely to develop which side-effects. Based on a Chinese analysis of both the therapeutic effects of Danazol and its side-effects, I believe Danazol works by causing blood vacuity in turn by weakening the spleen. Most endometriosis is due, at least in part, to blood stasis. If one reduces the total volume of blood, there will be less pressure and therefore less pain. In Chinese medicine, the common denominator between muscle cramps, hot flashes and flushing, and growth of facial hair is blood vacuity. As the blood becomes vacuous, so does the yin, including body fluids. This, in turn, allows yang or heat to get out of control. This heat then causes acne, vaginitis, and vulvitis. We have seen above that it is the spleen which initiates the creation of blood. One way to reduce the blood is to impair the function of the spleen. Since the spleen transforms and transports water, if it becomes dysfunctional, edema may occur. In Chinese medicine, obesity is an excess of dampness and phlegm due to spleen dysfunction. The spleen also governs the flesh according to Chinese medicine. Wasting of the flesh, meaning loss of a rounded figure, is due to the spleen's inability to nourish the flesh with adequate blood; therefore, decrease in breast size. Depending upon the pre-existing, constitutional condition of her spleen, an individual woman will react to Danazol either by becoming more damp and sodden or by becoming more dry and hot.

Since the blood is a vital, pure, nutritive substance according to Chinese medicine, its decrease forebodes accelerated aging in general and systemic debility. Women experience menopause or the exhaustion of their *tian gui* because of the inevitable exhaustion of their blood due to age. Danazol creates menopause by speeding up and creating this exhaustion. Traditional Chinese medicine finds this not only short-sighted and unwise but also fundamentally unacceptable. Rather, it destagnates the blood directly and then increases the creation and supply of this vital, nutritive substance. This then leads to retardation of the aging process and a general improvement in the health. It is not uncommon for women being treated for dysmenorrhea and infertility due to static and vacuous blood to report that their Chinese treatment not only successfully eliminated their major complaints but also caused their skin to become clearer, more youthful, and more moist, for their hair to become more lustrous, for their energy, sleep, and mood to all improve significantly, and for friends and relatives to report a generally rosy glow to their complexions and dispositions.

It is also a fact that hormone therapy, such as Danazol which causes pseudomenopause and Enovid, Norlutin, and Norlutate which cause pseudopregnancy, rarely cure moderate to severe endometriosis.[48] This is because moderate to severe endometriosis is more due to vacuity of the qi and blood due to the prolonged course of development of the condition. Therefore, further weakening of the blood would not make this situation any better and, in fact, in my opinion, would be likely to make it even worse.

Focus of Treatment

Chinese medicine only logically treats Chinese disease categories. However, that is not the same as saying Chinese medicine only treats Chinese people. Endometriosis is not a traditional Chinese disease category nor can it ever really become one. Since the only way to really make a confirmed diagnosis of endometriosis is by laparoscopy and laparotomy and since neither of these methods are included under any of the four methods of traditional Chinese diagnosis, Chinese medicine, in a semantic sense, does not treat endometriosis. What Chinese medicine does treat is painful menstruation (*tong jing*), menstruation which is too little or too large in volume (*yue jing guo shao* or *yue jing guo duo*), menstruation which is either too early, too late, or which occurs at no fixed schedule (*yue jing xian qi, yue jing hou qi,* or *yue jing xian hou wu ding qi*), vicarious menstruation or bleeding from orifices other than the vagina perimenstrually (*jing xing tu nu*), amenorrhea (*jing bi*), dysfunctional uterine bleeding (*beng lou*), premenstrual breast distention (and all other

---

[48] Ibid., p. 79 & 90

62

PMS symptoms, *jing xing ru fang zhang tong*), lower abdominal pain (*shao fu tong*), and infertility (*bu yun zheng*). And, Chinese medicine treats all of these effectively, cost-efficiently, and without iatrogenic side-effects.

Some women may ask, "You're treating my dysmenorrhea and lower abdominal pain, but how do I know my endometriosis will be cured?" This and similar questions come up all the time when treating Western patients with Chinese medicine. The answer to this question is not so simple and clear-cut as most of us would wish. It requires the patient to make a choice as to which description of their disease they feel is the most real for them. Endometriosis as a diagnosis is dependent upon laparoscopy and laparotomy. The rise in incidence of the *diagnosis* of endometriosis is, to a large measure, a function of the introduction and spread of these diagnostic techniques. Traditional Chinese medicine does not use these techniques and, in fact, feels these procedures themselves may actually exacerbate this condition, since the stress and surgical scar tissue, obstructing the free flow of the conception and penetrating vessels, only accentuate stagnation of the qi and blood stasis in the lower burner or pelvis.

On the other hand, Chinese medicine does have a complete and complex, differential diagnosis and rational theories concerning the disease mechanism for *all* the presenting signs and symptoms women experience when they have the Western disease endometriosis. What this means is that the Chinese doctor cannot, according to the logic of our own system, say we cure endometriosis, but we do routinely treat and cure all the signs and symptoms of endometriosis. The only way that we could say we cure endometriosis is if we suggested to our patients that, after having cured all their subjective signs and symptoms, they go and have a laparoscopy to see if their endometriosis is still there. However, I know of no traditional Chinese medical practitioner who would suggest such a thing.

For me, the bottom line is, if it looks like a pear, feels like a pear, and tastes like a pear, that's good enough for me. Or, a rose by any other name is still a rose. Western medicine has created the diagnosis of endometriosis based on its ability and penchant for looking surgically inside the body. Yet it cannot explain why endometrial cells are found outside the endometrium in some women. It has several theories but none are conclusive and none are enlightening on a human level. The Western theories about how and why endometriosis develops are all on a cellular and biochemical level about which the patient herself cannot do anything. The theories of Chinese medicine regarding the production of the disease conditions it recognizes all make very logical sense, are self-consistent and systematic, and also are enlightening and empowering from the human point of view. These Chinese theories of disease mechanism explain what everyday factors have led to the disease and immediately imply what the woman herself can do to rectify the situation. This empowers the patient, makes her life understandable, and ultimately endows her with increased wisdom about living life well. As such, I find the Chinese diagnoses of qi stagnation and blood stasis, accumulation of cold causing blood stasis, heat congestion with blood stasis, and qi and blood vacuity with blood stasis all *better* descriptions of what my patients are experiencing than the Western description endometriosis because they are ultimately more pragmatic on the human level.

This discussion may see like just so much unnecessary philosophizing, but, in my experience, those women who can understand this basic conceptual difference between Chinese and Western medicine and can wholeheartedly embrace the Chinese description of their condition are the ones who get the best results from Chinese medicine. Those women who ultimately believe in the Western description of their condition as being the really real one seldom stick with Chinese medicine long enough to get the best result. Such women try Chinese medicine as simply an alternative, empirical therapy. If it works, fine, but they are not interested in why and it better work quickly and without much personal change on their part. But Chinese medicine is not just something the physician does to one. It is a vision and philosophy of life. Those women who get the maximum results from Chinese medicine are those who both appreciate and embrace this philosophy of living. Ultimately, Chinese medicine is not just a collection of therapies but an education. This goes back to Sun Si-miao's opinion that the Superior Physician does not just treat disease but educates the intentions of society.

Duration of Therapy

Most menstrual problems, such as dysmenorrhea, menorrhagia, and early or late periods, can be treated by Chinese medicine within three to six months. However, the duration of therapy depends to some extent on the length of time the disease process has been in motion. I usually tell my patients to expect it to take at least one month of treatment for every year there has been some problem either with their period or in their pelvis in general. Thus, if a woman is thirty-five and she began having dysmenorrhea when she was twenty-three, she will probably need to take Chinese herbs in some form for at least a year.

Each period is a report card for the physician and the patient alike. The signs and symptoms surrounding each period are an accurate reflection of how the treatment is progressing. During the first month, the doctor makes his or her initial Chinese diagnosis. Although this is an educated and informed opinion, still it is a judgement and is subject to human fallibility. If the woman has come in early enough in her monthly cycle to get a full course of treatment and if the doctor's diagnosis and, therefore, treatment are correct, some improvement should be registered in the first period.

However, often women come in just before their period is about to begin and there is not enough time to do much meaningful therapy. In those cases, the next period is really the first course of treatment. Sometimes the practitioner's initial diagnosis is not one hundred percent correct. However, by seeing just how the period responds to whatever therapy was offered, the practitioner should be able to make their subsequent diagnosis and therapy even more accurate.

That means that it is often in the second month that major improvement is registered. Then, if all goes well and there are no complications, the third and fourth months should just be a kind of mopping-up operation. That means that in the third and fourth months, the practitioner tries to eliminate any residual or recalcitrant signs and symptoms. After all the major signs and symptoms are eliminated and the period is a full three to four day flow, painless, on time, with no particular premenstrual symptoms, a bright, fresh red and free from clots, most women will be suggested to take some mild form of Chinese herbs in pill, powder, or extract form. This is to consolidate the treatment and insure that the patient continues to move towards health.

Complications in treatment largely have to do with patient compliance. All too often in the West, patients go in and out of town on business or vacation right in the middle of their treatment. Chinese medicine is local medicine and requires a certain persistent regularity in the patient's therapy. Westerners are always, it seems, experiencing one upheaval or another—divorce, change of jobs, change of domicile, this crisis or that—and all such interruptions and upheavals generally set back the Chinese therapy. Chinese medicine requires a certain degree of commitment not generally required by Western medicine. If the patient does not do their relaxation, does not exercise, eats the wrong foods, forgets or cannot take their herbs on schedule, or cannot come in for acupuncture during the indicated times in their cycle, there is little the Chinese-style practitioner can do and all such vagaries result in the treatment taking longer.

After having undergone intensive Chinese herbal and acupuncture therapy for several cycles and after major irregularities surrounding the menstruation have been rectified, it is important that the patient continue working perseveringly with their stress reduction and relaxation, their exercise, and their diet. Qi stagnation as a Chinese diagnosis has a very high rate of recidivism. This is because it is due to stress and stress is endemic in our culture. Therefore, if a woman is not careful, she can easily fall back into all the old patterns which caused her problem in the first place. Depressive heat is only a complication of stagnant qi and so women with this diagnosis also tend to recreate it if they are not careful. Blood stasis due to cold generally can be treated quickly and does not tend to recur as easily as the two foregoing patterns. Vacuity of qi and blood likewise does not tend to recur if the woman watches her diet and does not overwork.

If any menstrual irregularities do recur, the woman should immediately return to her Chinese medical practitioner and undergo what is usually only a short course of therapy. Gong Ding-xian, a famous Qing dynasty physician, offered ten maxims to his patients, the third of which says,

> One should begin treatment at an early stage. At the beginning it is still simple. Whoever fails to be careful in hoarfrost will be surprised by solid ice.[49]

However, if a woman practices daily deep relaxation, keeps her stress under control and as minimal as possible, exercises every other day at least, and eats a sound, nutritious, easily digestible diet, then she should be able to maintain her health mostly by her own efforts.

Case Histories

The following case histories exemplify the traditional Chinese medical diagnosis and treatment of dysmenorrhea and other symptoms which are associated with the Western disease endometriosis.

Case I: The patient was 38 years old. Her main complaint was dysmenorrhea which had progressively gotten worse over the last ten years. It occurred on the first day of each period and the patient lost one day of work each month because of it. She had been treated by a Western MD with pain killers. The pain consisted of localized points of stabbing pain behind her sacrum. She also experienced pain on both sides of her abdomen just in front of her hip bones. Two nights before her period she experienced sciatic pain in the evenings with involuntary clenching of her toes. The dysmenorrhea itself started before the menstrual flow. The flow itself was scanty, dark, and clotty. Premenstrually the patient experienced emotional lability and breast distention with lumps. In addition, this patient also experienced lower abdominal bloating and bouts of flatulence from time to time. Her tongue, according to Chinese tongue diagnosis, was pale, a little swollen, scalloped along the edges, had a redder

---

[49] Gong Ding-xian, *Wen Ping Hui Chun*, trans. by Paul V. Unschuld, excerpted in *Medical Ethics in Imperial China*, U.C. Press, Berkeley, 1979, p. 72-73

than normal tip, and its coating was white and thicker than normal. Her Chinese pulse diagnosis was wiry on the right hand and wiry and thready on the left.

Based on the above signs and symptoms, my diagnosis was *tong jing* or dysmenorrhea due to stagnant qi and blood and liver/kidney yin vacuity with attendant premenstrual breast distention (*jing xing ru fang zhang tong*). I could tell she had blood stasis because of her fixed, stabbing pain, and clotty discharge. I could tell she had liver depression and qi stagnation because of her wiry pulse, premenstrual and lower abdominal distention, flatulence, emotional lability, and dark menstrual discharge. Liver blood/kidney yin vacuity was suggested by the thready left pulse, the scant menstrual volume, the premenstrual sciatica with the clenching of toes in the evening, and the pale tongue with the redder than normal tip. In addition, her somewhat fluted, scalloped tongue also suggested that her spleen qi had become weak and was not transporting and transforming body fluids properly due to encroachment by the liver (liver invading the spleen). In other words, each of the patient's signs and symptoms led me to a very individualized and comprehensive diagnosis. None of the signs and symptoms were meaningless, unexplainable, or illogical according to Chinese medical theory.

The patient, like many such, initiated Chinese treatment just before the expected onset of her pain. Therefore, I was only able to give her one acupuncture treatment and only two days of herbs. When the patient got her period, all the pain was concentrated on the right side of her abdomen which was quite different from her previous experience. However, its intensity was no less.

The next cycle, the patient began herbal and acupuncture therapy one week before the expected due date of her period as I had suggested. This time she took Chinese herbal medicine through the first day of her period and received one acupuncture treatment every other day for three treatments. Her period came on time with no real dysmenorrhea. All she experienced was a little low back pain and twinges of sciatica.

The next cycle, the patient only took herbs and did not receive any acupuncture. Again she started the herbs one week before the expected onset of her period. Again she had no real dysmenorrhea. Her menstrual discharge was fuller, not so dark, and was without clots. Her only complaint this time was still some twinges of sciatica. This meant her blood stasis had been eliminated. Liver blood/kidney yin vacuity takes times to rectify since these vital substances are only built back up slowly over time. Therefore, I prescribed a Chinese herbal patient medicine in pill form for sciatica due to liver/kidney vacuity which the woman took for several months to consolidate the therapeutic result.

Case II: This patient was also 38 years old. She complained of pain at her right waist which had persisted for one year. It had begun as pain only at ovulation and during her period but was now continuous. Her period was regular at 28 days. She experienced lots of cramping, worse in the last year, and her discharge was dark red and clotty. The pain was only crampy, not stabbing, and lasted the twenty-four hours of the first day of her period. Premenstrually, she experienced temporal headaches, breast soreness and lumps, and some emotional lability which was getting worse. Her tongue was pale and brownish with a yellowish-white coating to the rear. Her pulse was fine and wiry.

This woman's Chinese diagnosis was lower abdominal pain (*shao fu tong*), dysmenorrhea, and premenstrual breast pain due to liver depression and qi stagnation and blood vacuity and incipient blood stasis. Her wiry pulse, brownish tongue, premenstrual headaches along the course of the gallbladder channel, breast soreness, and crampy menstrual pain all suggested liver depression and qi stagnation. Her pale tongue and thready pulse indicated blood vacuity. And the menstrual clots but no stabbing pain indicated that blood stasis was in the process of forming but was as yet minimal and insubstantial.

This woman also initiated Chinese therapy just before the onset of her period. Therefore, I could only administer a single acupuncture treatment. This resulted in relieving all the premenstrual cramps and her premenstrual headache although the cramps with her period were the same. The next month I was able to administer Chinese herbal medicine beginning one week before the onset of her period and gave her one more acupuncture treatment which completely eliminated her dysmenorrhea. Unfortunately, this woman did not understand the importance of continuing with her therapy after the disappearance of her major complaint and so she stopped Chinese medicine at that point.

Case III: The patient was 41 years old. Two years previously she had had an ovary removed which had become the size of a grapefruit. At that time she had been diagnosed as suffering from endometriosis. That surgery succeeded in relieving her dysmenorrhea but since then she experienced increasingly severe premenstrual emotional lability beginning at ovulation, menorrhagia or profuse bleeding with her periods, bad perimenstrual headaches accompanied by sensitivity to light, and premenstrual breast distention. These symptoms were accompanied by extreme fatigue which did not improve until four to six days after her period. She complained of being edematous by the end of each day, was stiff in her joints in the morning, woke in the early hours of the morning each night, and felt jittery and wired. Her gums bled and her bowel movements alternated from being constipated to loose. Her chest was very tight, she was thirsty, her memory was becoming poor, and she had lots of gas. Her cycle fluctuated from 26—29 days with the menorrhagia starting on the second day and lasting two days. Her tongue was pale, fluted, and trembling and her tongue coating was thin, white, and slightly dry. Her pulse was fast, wiry, and slippery on the right and fast, wiry, and fine on the left.

My Chinese diagnosis of this woman was menorrhagia (*yue jing guo duo*) and premenstrual breast distention due to a combination of depressive liver heat and qi and blood vacuity. In this case, liver depression and qi stagnation had transformed into depressive heat. The liver qi evidenced itself by the breast distention, tight chest, flatulence, constipation, slightly irregular periods, wiry pulse, and emotional lability. The fact that this had transformed into heat was evidenced by the bleeding gums, menorrhagia, and fast pulse. The headaches were a combination of replete liver qi and heat plus liver blood vacuity. The blood vacuity was due to the menorrhagia (liver not storing the blood) and it

70

was indicated by the pale tongue and fine pulse on the left, bad memory, and sensitivity to light. Again, because of the liver invading the spleen, this woman experienced edema (spleen not transporting and transforming liquids correctly), loose stools, and extreme fatigue. This spleen qi vacuity also contributed to the menorrhagia (qi not holding the blood within its vessels). The trembling tongue showed that there was serious vacuity of both the qi and blood and the slippery quality of the right pulse and slightly dry tongue coating showed that liquids were not being transported and transformed.

In this case, the first thing necessary to do was to supplement the qi and blood and to strengthen and regulate the spleen. This would automatically help to control and relax the liver. This patient commenced treatment just at the end of her period when she was most fatigued and having a bad headache. Two packets of herbs took away the headache, helped her fatigue, and enabled her to sleep soundly through the night. She took herbs continuously through this whole first cycle. At mid-cycle her breasts became sore and I added ingredients to her formula to relieve that, which they did. Also her edema was relieved. She came in for one acupuncture treatment, but because of her very busy and stressful schedule, she could not come in for more. She had no other PMS symptoms until one day before her period when all her symptoms returned.

The next month, this woman took herbs from mid-cycle through the onset of her period. Her premenstrual symptoms were minimal, a little breast discomfort and a little grouchiness. Her flatulence had worsened and this time her period came two days early and she had dysmenorrhea for 12-14 hours. However, her bleeding was not especially profuse. This all indicated that we had succeeded in supplementing her qi and blood which had then aggravated temporarily her liver qi and heat. This then caused the dysmenorrhea and the period's coming two days early. After her period was over. I gave her herbs for two days to strengthen her heart and kidneys based on the famous Qing dynasty gynecologist Fu Qing-zhu's opinion that a stuck and over-heated liver can be remedied by supplementing these two viscera because of five phase energetics. This helped this patient sleep even more soundly.

71

Again, since we had treated this woman's main complaint, menorrhagia, she discontinued Chinese therapy at this point. Because she never did understand the necessity of deep relaxation, stress reduction, and regular exercise, I doubt whether her situation remained satisfactory. Unfortunately, because of Westerner's conceptual habits regarding health care established by Western medicine, many similar patients fail to follow Chinese medicine as far as it could potentially take them.

Case IV: This woman came for treatment when she was 32. Her major complaint was a lengthened menstrual cycle of 45 days. She experienced some cramping during the first day. She had a six day flow followed by three days of spotting. Her discharge was dark red and gelatinous but not clotty. She had diarrhea each month for one day at the onset of her period. She also had *mittelschmerz* every other month. She used to have premenstrual breast and lower abdominal distention and facial edema, but since she had eliminated sugar from her diet, these had been relieved. However, if she ate sugar, her premenstrual signs and symptoms returned. Stress tended to delay her period and the patient reported that stress was continuous in her life. Also before her period, she would get acne around her mouth. Her tongue had a red rim with orangey, slightly fluted sides. There was a centerline cleft with yellow, thorn-like fur. Otherwise, her tongue was dry in the center with a whitish-yellowish coating. Her pulse was simply wiry.

This woman's Chinese diagnosis was delayed menstruation (*yue jing hou qi*) due to liver qi, spleen vacuity, and a tendency to develop liver/stomach heat before each period. The liver qi was evidenced by the delayed period and cramping and the wiry pulse. The liver qi failed to mobilize the blood for expulsion in a timely manner because it was hung-up. However, there was no blood stasis. Instead, her spleen was weak and this was why sugar made her symptoms worse, since a vacuous spleen allows the liver to become all the more replete. The diarrhea at the onset of menstruation was also due to spleen vacuity. But, when the liver is replete and the spleen is vacuous, the stomach can get hot. This was indicated in this patient by her premenstrual, perioral acne, her increased premenstrual sexual desire, her gelatinous discharge as if the blood had been stewed, and her dry tongue with the centerline fissure within which were thorns of yellow fur.

Since this woman did not suffer from marked pain, her professional Chinese treatment consisted of only herbal medicine and not acupuncture. She took Chinese herbal medicine in pill form for several months. This shortened her cycle to approximately thirty days at which point the blood became less gelatinous. However, at this point the patient came under even more stress by going back to school. Her PMS got worse, she developed heartburn, irritability, flank pain, a tight chest, a voracious appetite and thirst, breast distention, a distended lower abdomen, and fatigue. Although her period was no longer overdue, her liver qi had transformed into depressive heat thus aggravating her stomach heat and again weakening her spleen. The patient had to be switched to Chinese herbal medicine in decoction which then brought all her symptoms under control in six days.

Case V: This last case history is of a 25 year old, recent graduate from law school. Her sister called asking me to come right over in order to treat her extreme dysmenorrhea. When I arrived, I found her crying and sweating curled up on the bed. Her face was flushed, she felt nauseous, and her cramps were extreme. Her pulse was tight and retarded. I administered emergency acupuncture and within ten minutes her pain began to subside. After twenty minutes, she was greatly relieved and experiencing only minimal discomfort. Shortly after that, she fell asleep and napped for a couple of hours.

A couple of months later, she came to see me in my office. Her major complaint was premenstrual nosebleeds and continued dysmenorrhea. Her face was still flushed, she felt hot often, her menstrual blood was bright red and voluminous, and her pulse was wiry and rapid. My diagnosis was *jing xing tu nu* or what is called vicarious menstruation, perimenstrual bleeding through a non-vaginal orifice, plus dysmenorrhea due to depressive liver heat. The depressive heat was due to over-eating hot, spicy foods (in southern Colorado) and the stress of her new job. Several packets of herbs eliminated the premenstrual epistaxis. But because this woman lived six or more hours drive away, all I could do is send her herbs from time to time.

Several months later, she again developed premenstrual nosebleeds and again Chinese herbal medicine put a stop to them. Then a year more went by and the patient visited Boulder again. At this point, she was having extreme menorrhagia likewise due to heat. I treated her with acupuncture and we stopped the bleeding and again I sent her herbs for some time to consolidate the effect. A year after that, again she developed menorrhagia and again we were able to treat it. After that, I lost contact.

This case history points up the fact that Chinese medicine is local medicine. It does not work well at a distance since a great deal of adjustment, up-dating, and feedback are required for really best, long-term results. This woman resorted to Chinese medicine as a symptomatic treatment on an as-needed basis. And Chinese medicine worked each time. However, this is only the beginning of Chinese medicine's potential health-promoting benefits.

INFERTILITY

Female infertility is called *Bu Yun Zheng* in traditional Chinese medicine. This literally means "no pregnancy condition". In China today, it is defined as "failure to conceive after over three years of marriage even though both parties are (otherwise seemingly) healthy, or failure to conceive for several years after the first delivery."[50] The editors of *Progress in Infertility* open on page one with the statement:

The number of married couples (in America) unable to conceive has climbed from 15 percent to 18 to 20 percent in the past decade... Increasingly, the infertile couple may both be highly productive members of society, successful in all but their ability to conceive.[51]

Drs. Behrman, Kistner, and Patton go on to state that, "A different American lifestyle has contributed to the increased number of infertility patients seen by the physician in this decade."[52]

In traditional Chinese, Confucian society, failure to have children and especially sons was regarded as a personal disaster of the highest magnitude. Without sons, there was no one to make sacrifices to the ancestors and so one's immortality was cut off or impoverished. Therefore, Chinese medicine as an expression of Chinese society placed great emphasis on the treatment of both male sterility and female infertility. However, as with all other pathologies, Chinese medicine diagnoses and treats infertility without expensive lab

---

[50] Song & Yu, op.cit., p. 131

[51] *Progress In Infertility*, op.cit., p. 1

[52] Ibid., p. 1

tests or invasive and iatrogenic procedures. Rather, it relies on centuries of acute observation and its time-tested, systematic categorization of the constitutional signs and symptoms infertile women almost invariably present.

Traditional Chinese doctors could not and cannot see the ovum with our naked eyes. Therefore, Chinese medicine's description of conception is different from Western medicine's. Chinese doctors could see the ejaculate of men and knew that men had to ejaculate in women before the woman could become pregnant. But the only thing, other than vaginal mucous and babies, they could see coming out of women's vaginas was blood. They also knew that before the onset and after the cessation of menstruation, women are infertile and also that during pregnancy, menstruation ceases. Therefore, traditional doctors throughout Asia came to the conclusion that conception takes place when the sperm from the man unites with the blood of the woman in her uterus or fetal palace. Chang Huang, writing in the sixteenth century, expresses this classical Chinese view: "When the father's semen and the mother's blood contact each other, they unite and congeal to become the fetus in the womb."[53]

The entire diagnosis and treatment of infertility in traditional Chinese medicine is an extension of this basic belief. Anything that might cause this blood to be insufficient might cause infertility. Likewise, anything that might cause blockage or stagnation of the blood's ability to flow freely to and through the womb might also cause infertility. Since menstruation is the clearest and most obvious indication of the quantity, quality, and patency of the blood, Zhu Dan-xi, one of the Four Great Masters of Internal medicine of the Jin/Yuan dynasties, said, "In order to cure infertility, the first important thing is to adjust the menstruation."[54] By adjusting the menstruation, Zhu meant treating

---

[53] Chang Huang, *Du Shu Pian,* trans by Paul V. Unschuld, excerpted in *Introductory Readings in Classical Chinese Medicine*, Kluwer Academic Publishers, Dordrecht, Boston, London, 1988, p. 57

[54] Zhu Dan-xi quoted by Cong Chun-yi, "Personal Experiences in the Treatment of Infertility", trans. by Yong Huai-yuan & Bob Flaws, *Blue Poppy Essays, 1988*, Blue

any menstrual pathology, such as early or late menstruation, hyper or hypomenorrhea, dysmenorrhea, premenstrual breast distention, or amenorrhea. Since Chinese medicine treats all of these conditions quite well, it likewise treats female infertility with a high degree of success.

Basically, the blood collecting and circulating through the uterus can be either insufficient or blocked because of two broad categories of disease factors. These two categories are 1) congenital physiological deficiency and 2) acquired pathological phenomena. The first category traditionally includes five congenital anatomical abnormalities, such as malformation of the uterus, which make pregnancy impossible. The second category describes imbalances causing infertility which are not congenital but which a woman might develop over time. This second category is then subdivided into six basic disease mechanisms resulting in infertility. In comparing five different Chinese differential diagnoses for infertility, the main patterns of disharmony accounting for this condition in women are:

1) Kidney vacuity
2) Liver depression qi stagnation
3) Blood vacuity

4) Cold uterus
5) Depressive heat
6) Phlegm dampness[55]

Although these six disease mechanisms account for the majority of cases of female infertility, in individual patients, various of these factors may combine to form more complicated, idiosyncratic scenarios. Also, several of these patterns have subdivisions which must also be distinguished.

Poppy Press, Boulder, CO, 1988, p. 38

[55] The five sources consulted were: Song & Yu, op.cit.; Han Bai-ling, op.cit.; Lu, Henry, *Doctor's Manual of Chinese Medical Diet*, Vol.II,Chinese Foundation of Natural Health, Vancouver, BC, 1981, p. 204; *Fu Ke Zheng Zhi (Proven Gynecological Treatments)*, Sun Jiu-sheng, ed., Hebei People's Press, Shijiashuang, PRC, 1983, 143-147; Qiu Mao-lian & Su Xin-ming, The Nanjing Seminars Transcript, *Journal of Chinese Medicine*, Hove, UK, 1985, p. 13-19

Kidney Vacuity

As mentioned above in discussing endometriosis, there are three viscera which participate in creating the blood. These are the heart, the spleen, and the kidneys. The kidneys provide *jing* or essence to form the essential substrate of the blood. If this kidney *jing* is vacuous or insufficient, blood cannot be produced up to normal volume. This *jing* is of two types. The first is congenital. We are each endowed with a certain quantity and quality of this congenital essence (*xian tian zhi jing*) at the moment of conception and this cannot be augmented or modified. However, it is slowly used as we live our life and natural death comes when we have completely burnt through this original endowment.

The second type of *jing* is called acquired essence (*hou tian zhi jing*). It is manufactured from the surplus qi and blood manufactured through digestion. If there is any qi and blood manufactured during the day which is not consumed by that day's activities, this can be converted into acquired essence to be stored in the kidneys while we sleep. This acquired essence shores up and bolsters our congenital essence. When it is strong and abundant, relatively little congenital essence is combusted. However, if through fatigue, stress, poor diet, bad digestion, poor sleep, overstimulation, and sexual excess we either fail to create acquired essence or use it too precipitously, we will exhaust whatever acquired essence we do have and then begin consuming our congenital essence.

If either we are born with insufficient congenital essence or we use up or fail to make acquired essence, our blood production will also be insufficient. And, if the blood is insufficient, conception cannot take place, or, if per chance it does, the fetus will not be nourished properly and miscarriage is likely.

Kidney function is spoken of as kidney qi and some Chinese texts talk of kidney qi vacuity when discussing infertility. However, kidney function, in Chinese medicine, is subdivided into kidney yin and kidney yang. Kidney yin is the *jing* essence and the substantial aspect of the kidney. Kidney yang is its active, warm, functional part. Therefore, some authors describe kidney yang vacuity infertility patterns and kidney yin vacuity infertility patterns. Since yin and yang are mutually interdependent and interpromoting, if either is vacuous, kidney *jing* may also be compromised and thus the blood as well. As a further complication, if kidney yin becomes vacuous, the yang of the body or its functional warmth will begin to burn out of control like a smoldering fire. This low-grade but persistent pathogenic Heat tends to flush up to the liver and the heart, eventually affecting their functions. This heat exhausts or evaporates the blood in these two important viscera, one of which helps to create the blood (the heart) and one of which stores the blood (the liver). Therefore, not only is the essence substrate insufficient for catalyzing the creation of new blood, but the blood that has already been created is even further exhausted.

The signs and symptoms of kidney yang vacuity infertility include persistent low back pain, weakness, and "cold" pain, weak knees, cold feet, polyuria with voluminous, clear urine, nocturia, watery leukorrhea, possible menorrhagia with a thin, dilute discharge, fatigue, fear of cold, persistent day-break diarrhea, tinnitus, palpitations, dizziness, a pale tongue with a white coating, and a deep, slow, weak pulse. Kidney yang vacuity is not so frequently met with amongst young Western adults. When it is seen, it is usually due to extreme abuse of drugs, such as cocaine, or as part of a more complicated, chronic scenario involving the spleen. If it is due to congenital weakness, it may be impossible to correct. If it is due to exhaustion, sexual excess, prolonged disease, or drugs, it can be treated with Chinese herbal medicine, rest and relaxation, a warm, nourishing diet, and moxibustion.

The signs and symptoms of kidney yin vacuity infertility are weak lower back, sore knees, polyuria but with scant, darkish urine, tinnitus, palpitations, insomnia in the early morning hours, fatigue, nocturia, a redder than normal tongue with scant coating, and a thready pulse. If yin vacuity results in the production of an uncontrollable vacuity heat or fire, there will be feverish feelings in the hands, feet, and center of the chest, flushing of the cheeks when exhausted or in the evenings, night sweats, hot flashes, vaginal inflammation, possible burning urination, mental unrest and agitation, an even redder tongue with scant, yellow coating, and a floating, fine, and fast pulse.

In terms of menstruation, kidney yin vacuity can cause early or late periods, metrorrhagia or breakthrough bleeding, or amenorrhea. Kidney yin vacuity can be due to drugs, excessive sex, excessive activity and stimulation, persistent inflammatory conditions, stress, emotional upset, coffee, tea, smoking, insufficient rest and sleep, and a poor, non-nourishing diet.

Kidney yin vacuity is more commonly met with amongst young and middle-aged Western adults. However, it is rarely encountered as a pure pattern in women complaining of infertility. Rather, it is often a complicating factor in women with other, simultaneous and interrelated patterns, such as liver qi, liver blood vacuity, and spleen dampness. If yang is activity and yin is substance or fuel, yin vacuity is due to hyperactivity too rapidly consuming our form or substance. This could be an apt metaphor for describing our culture as a whole. Since our yin is consumed in the act of living in any case, some element of kidney yin vacuity often colors cases of women with infertility in their late thirties and early forties.

Kidney yin vacuity infertility can be treated successfully by Chinese herbal medicine and acupuncture. However, it demands deep relaxation, a nutritious diet from which acquired essence can be created and stored, life-style modifications to reduce stress and overstimulation, and complete abstinence from drugs and stimulants, such as coffee, nicotine, and alcohol. Because this pattern results in frenetic activity and a pervasive restlessness, this pattern is often difficult to treat because people with this scenario have a hard time slowing down. When they do, they become aware of how frenetic and jittery they are and it is easier, although more debilitating, to give into this frenetic qi and keep moving. As a result, they are often impatient, irresolute, and indecisive. They cannot wait for the herbs, diet, and deep relaxation to work. They want results now and if results are not immediately forthcoming with one system, they will search out another which promises a quicker fix. Unfortunately, the kidney yin, as the root of all yin of the body, is only regenerated slowly from whatever surplus is created and stored each day. Therefore, its recuperation is, especially at first, very slow. With this particular pattern of infertility, the woman's motto should be, "Slow and steady wins the race." Paradoxically, these are just the women who most acutely feel their biological clock ticking and who are the most impatient for results. This then becomes a Catch-22.

Liver Depression & Qi Stagnation

We have already discussed above the mechanics of this pattern. Since the qi moves the blood and since the uterus is irrigated by the liver, impatency of liver qi will tend to retard the blood flow in the uterus. This then prevents or blocks conception from taking place even though there might be sufficient blood otherwise. In terms of menstruation, liver depression and qi stagnation often result in late, irregular, or absent periods, dysmenorrhea, and premenstrual depression, emotionality, and breast distention, lumps, and pain. Liver depression and qi stagnation over time can also lead to blood stasis, which is an even worse blockage of the uterus. Because of the numerous interrelationships of the qi and blood and the liver and other viscera, liver qi usually presents as only part of a more complicated scenario. Very commonly, women will have liver qi, blood vacuity, and spleen vacuity and/or dampness all at the same time with the proportions of each varying with the stages in the menstrual cycle.

Interestingly, breast distention was not discussed much in the classic Chinese literature, mostly due to modesty and sexual reticence. However, the one place it does appear is in discussions of infertility.[56] This is so much so that premenstrual breast distention is almost synonymous with infertility in the classical literature. My experience as a clinician is that the incidence and severity of premenstrual breast distention rises as a woman moves through her thirties and into her forties, which exactly corresponds to the statistical decrease in fertility which occurs at the same time. And, when treating this

---

[56] Zhu Xiao-nan, anthologized in *Shang Hai Lao Zhong Yi Jing Yan Xuan Bian (A Collection of Shanghai Old Masters' Clinical Experiences)*, Shanghai Science & Technology Press, Shanghai, 1984, a precis of which appears in English in *Free and Easy*, op.cit., p. 97-107

type of infertility, great attention is paid to the eventual remedying of this symptom. When the woman's period is regular and she no longer has any premenstrual breast complaints, she should then be fertile according to Chinese medicine.[57] The relationship between the uterus, the liver, and the breasts is due to an internal branch of the liver meridian running to the nipple and an internal branch of the penetrating vessel also running to the breast. In addition, the breast is more superficially irrigated by the stomach channel which connects with the penetrating vessel and therefore the liver and the uterus in the groin region.

Because liver qi can be involved with so many other related, complicating patterns, the textbook signs and symptoms of this pure pattern are somewhat misleading since they are seldom encountered, at least not here in the West, in their pure form. However, besides premenstrual breast distention, they include lower abdominal bloating, menstrual cramping, constipation and/or diarrhea, irritability, depression, emotional lability, tightness of the chest and therefore frequent sighing, headaches, and a wiry pulse.

Liver qi becomes congested whenever a person experiences a blockage in their life. Whenever our qi cannot flow freely, whether that be inside us mentally and emotionally or outside us in our daily activities, this may result in liver qi. Therefore, stress, frustration, and repression are the main causes of liver qi. It is not, primarily, a dietary problem, although over-eating heavy, hard to digest, greasy, fatty, oily foods can aggravate it, as can coffee, alcohol, and spicy, hot foods. Qi stagnation is due to stress and stress is endemic within our society. If one travels to a developing country and lives among the people, one quickly realizes how pressurized, stressful, and frustrating our Western life-style is. This is exactly the "different American life-style" which Drs. Behrman, Kistner, and Patton alluded to at the beginning of this section.

The good news is that Chinese herbal medicine and acupuncture coupled with deep relaxation and stress reduction, aerobic exercise, and proper diet can eliminate liver qi stagnation at least to the point of allowing conception and

---

[57] Ibid., p. 103-105

pregnancy. Because our stress is so continuous and pervasive, liver qi has a very high rate of recidivism or recurrence, but still, it can usually be rectified to at least treat infertility. That is *if* the woman is willing and able to modify her life-style and practice daily, deep relaxation. And there is one further complication when attempting to treat this pattern in Western women in their late thirties. Each month is an emotional crisis. There is a kind of deadline and the occurrence of each period signals both a defeat and the loss of precious time. Therefore, the approach of each period is attended with fear and dread. Then, when the period comes and it turns out the woman is not pregnant, once again this fear and dread give way to frustration, anger, depression, impatience, and hopelessness which all only cause more liver depression qi stagnation.

Therefore, with women with this pattern of infertility, it is imperative that they adopt their Chinese treatment as much for their own better, over-all health as for conceiving a baby. If the woman becomes totally goal-oriented on conceiving, this will, according to the logic of Chinese medicine, directly mitigate against conception. In the over-whelming majority of such cases, there will be some menstrual irregularity or breast distention at the least, and the woman is advised to recognize that these irregularities are important early warning signals which should be treated regardless of attempting to become a mother. Although they may seem inconsequential when compared with the woman's yearning and need to become a mother, still she should try to recognize that if these irregularities are not corrected, they will lead, in time, to more serious and even life-threatening problems. Honora Lee Wolfe, in *The Breast Connection*, describes the complex inter-relationships between the liver, breasts, and other organs and bodily functions and shows clearly how premenstrual breast distention may eventually become breast cancer.[58] Therefore, the woman owes it to herself to seek treatment *first* for herself and to continue treatment for herself until these irregularities are corrected. Then, when they are corrected, she will also find that she is fertile, since fertility is nothing other than the expression of full and unimpeded vitality in a woman.

---

[58] Wolfe, Honora Lee, *The Breast Connection, A Laywoman's Guide to the Treatment of Breast Diseases by Chinese Medicine,* Blue Poppy Press, Boulder, CO, 1989

Typically, liver depression qi stagnation infertility can be reversed in from three to nine months. Whether it takes three or nine months depends upon the patient's compliance and perseverance with the total program. If she can relax deeply once every day as a practice and then also throughout the day as a style of being, if she exercises, eats right, and receives acupuncture and Chinese herbal medicine all on schedule, my experience is that the results will be there. The following statistics on the traditional Chinese treatment of infertility are quite impressive. Of twenty women treated for premenstrual breast distention and infertility with various of their cases complicated by spleen vacuity, blood vacuity, kidney vacuity, cold accumulation in the penetrating and conception vessels, and flaring of liver fire, thirteen became pregnant. A further six women experienced subjective improvement in their symptoms but did not conceive within the time frame of the study which only spanned several months. And only one woman neither conceived nor experienced any relief in her other symptoms.[59]

The standard guiding herbal formula for the treatment of liver qi infertility is called Xiao Yao San. *Xiao Yao* means free and easy. *San* means powder but it also means dispersal. The name then is a double entendre. It means free and easy dispersal. When Chinese doctors talk about treating liver qi, they often use the word *shu* or dredge. The image is of dredging a silted-in river. If one removes the blockage, then all that is necessary is to stand back and allow the river to flow wherever it will. One needn't try to push the river. The *Nei Jing*, the most ancient Chinese medical classic, describes how one should act to benefit their liver:

> (One who desires to order their life in accordance with this season, the spring, the season of the liver according to five phase theory) goes to bed at night and rises early. They move through the court with long strides. Their hair hangs freely down the back of their neck; their (physical) appearance is relaxed. This way they cause their mind to grow. To bring to life, not to kill; to give, not take away; to reward, not to punish; these are (the actions) in accord with the qi

---

[59] Zhu, *Free and Easy*, op.cit., p. 103

which (embraces humanity) in the spring; this is the (correct) way to support the generation (of all things).[60]

Zorba the Greek would have said, "Dance."

Blood Vacuity

We have seen just how important enough blood is to conception according to Chinese medicine. Therefore, a major cause of infertility is due to insufficient blood. If kidney essence is sufficient, this mostly means blood vacuity due to the spleen and heart not creating the blood out of the digestate. The spleen's job is to send the pure part of the liquids of digestion up to the heart to be turned red. This is called *zhuo gui xin*, the gathering of the liquid part of the digestate at the heart to become blood. Therefore, if either the spleen or heart are too weak to do their job, blood cannot be made. Also the blood cannot be made if the spleen is not supplied with the proper nutrients to send up to the heart.

Both the heart and the spleen's function *vis à vis* blood production is susceptible to emotional disturbance. If the heart is "broken" or longing, it cannot create blood even if the spleen is sound. As for the spleen, its function is impaired by worry. Therefore, it is important to avoid indulging in these two emotions if one's blood is deficient. However, in most cases of blood vacuity I encounter in the West, faulty diet plays the largest part.

Over-eating raw fruits and vegetables, chilled, iced, and frozen foods and drinks, and drinking too many cold juices, are all contemporary Western causes for blood vacuity. Among certain segments of the Western population into health foods, not eating enough animal protein is also a contributing cause of blood vacuity. As we have seen when discussing diet under endometriosis,

---

[60] *Nei Jing*, translated by Paul V. Unschuld, excerpted in *Introductory Readings in Classical Chinese Medicine*, op.cit., p. 106

the process of digestion is one of warm transformation. The spleen/stomach must turn all food into 100° degree soup. Cooking one's food is predigestion and substantially increases its digestibility and, therefore, its net value. Raw fruits and vegetables tend to be cool or cold and dampening. This then impedes spleen function, resulting in poor production of qi and blood. If one wants to increase their production of blood, they should eat freshly cooked food which is easily digestible. This should include fresh vegetables, grains, legumes, especially black beans and black soy beans, and some animal protein. A rice, black bean, and vegetable broth made with a marrow bone is a very good sample meal for creating blood. In small portions, animal flesh is considered very "compassionate" to the human body and nourishes yin of which the blood is a part. Although raw vegetables seem to be more "alive", they are hard to digest and do not result in the same substantial net gain as do *lightly* cooked, fresh foods.

The signs and symptoms of blood vacuity are pallor, dizziness, blurred vision, night blindness, palpitations, insomnia, headaches, numbness in the fingers and toes, muscle cramps, a pale tongue, and fine pulse. In terms of menstruation, it tends to be scant, late, or entirely absent. However, these signs and symptoms are most often compounded with signs and symptoms relating to the liver, heart, spleen, and kidneys and to the qi. Seldom is blood vacuity met with as a pure pattern. Most often it complicates liver qi patterns, spleen/heart and liver/kidney dual vacuities, and spleen damp patterns.

Once again, the good news is that Chinese medicine treats blood vacuity quite well. In Chinese herbal medicine, there is a whole class of ingredients which specifically nourish or build the blood, Dang Gui or Radix Angelicae Sinensis being the most famous. Usually it takes several months to build the blood in an infertile woman. However, she will immediately know this is happening because her periods will become a fuller, fresher red and, if they are overdue, they will come closer and closer to a twenty-eight day schedule. Acupuncture can also catalyze the creation of blood, but there must be the correct diet supplying the building blocks for acupuncture to be effective. When one combines acupuncture, Chinese blood supplementing herbs, and a good, nourishing diet together, one can build the blood very effectively.

The lay reader is cautioned to remember that blood vacuity is a professional Chinese diagnostic category or pattern of disharmony. A woman may be anemic according to Western medicine and not be blood vacuous according to Chinese medicine and vice versa, although often blood vacuity and anemia do go together. In any case, Chinese medicine does recognize, diagnose, and treat blood vacuity. In the process, the woman's skin, hair, eyes, sleep, energy, and equipoise will all improve.

Cold Uterus

In Chinese medicine, life is warmth. If the womb or uterus is too cold, life cannot arise. In addition, cold tends to restrict the flow of qi and blood just as it freezes water. Pathogenic cold can effect the uterus in either of two ways. The first is vacuity cold.

A cold uterus due to vacuity mostly refers to yang vacuity of the kidneys. The kidney yang is the root of all yang in the body and, in particular, is the source of warmth in the pelvis or lower burner. We have already discussed kidney yang vacuity infertility above under the general heading of kidney vacuity. Since the kidney yang and spleen yang are mutually interdependent, long-term spleen vacuity can eventually lead to or complicate kidney yang vacuity and vice versa. Therefore, in some cases, one may find spleen/kidney yang vacuity. When this happens, both spleen and kidneys not only lack sufficient warmth to keep life's activities up to par, but they also fail to transport and transform fluids properly. This leads to the further complication of this scenario by the accumulation of dampness. Therefore, some Chinese gynecology texts identify a pattern of cold damp congelation and stagnation infertility.[61]

A cold uterus can also be due to a replete accumulation of cold in the uterus. That means that cold as a positive entity somehow has either invaded or been

---

[61] *Fu Ke Zheng Zhi*, op.cit., p. 144

incorporated into the body and, in the case of infertility, has lodged specifically in the womb. This can happen either by invasion of external pathogenic cold into the uterus from the outside environment or by over-eating iced, chilled, and frozen foods and liquids. In the first case, cold can invade the uterus through the lower gate (the vaginal meatus), during menstruation or during or directly after childbirth. In both instances, the body must open in order to discharge the menstruate and the baby and later the lochia. When the body opens for such discharge, it is also susceptible to invasion by external pathogens. Sixty or seventy years ago even in the West, women knew not to get chilled or go swimming during menstruation. I have also seen women who apparently were invaded by external pathogenic cold during surgical procedures, such as D & Cs. And fashion also may play its part. Wearing miniskirts during the winter and especially during menstruation may also permit easy access to the womb by invading cold.

Replete cold may also be due to eating chilled, frozen, and iced foods and liquids. Americans are habituated to eating and drinking chilled things due to universal access to refrigeration. However, eating too many chilled and frozen foods is extremely deleterious to the long-term health and, in particular, can cause blood stasis in the uterus due to cold congelation. These foods are even more harmful to healthy menstruation if they are eaten just before or at the onset of menstruation when, in fact, they are often craved. Ice cream, chilled sodas, chilled fruit juices, frozen yogurt, etc. are often craved by premenstrual women. This is because their livers and stomachs are hot and replete, thus making their spleens vacuous. The spleen craves the sweet flavor when vacuous and so such women crave sugar and carbohydrates. The cold temperature symptomatically allays the heat. But these foods are all also very damp and so again there is the complicated scenario of cold and dampness obstructing the uterus, only this time it is replete rather than vacuity cold.

The signs and symptoms of a cold uterus include protracted but scant menstrual discharge mixed with dark clots, dark menstrual blood, lower abdominal pain relieved by warmth, a thin, white tongue coating, and a deep, sunken pulse. If due to yang vacuity, there will be signs and symptoms of kidney dysfunction, such as polyuria, nocturia, low back and knee pain, and cold feet. If there is complicating dampness, there may also be polyuria, nocturia, and leukorrhea. If both kidney yang and spleen yang are vacuous, there will be chronic loose stools or daybreak diarrhea and generalized chill. In cases of vacuity cold, there will also be fatigue, but not in replete cases.

Happily, of all the causes of menoxenia (abnormal menstruation) and infertility, cold stagnation in the uterus is one of the easiest to treat with Chinese medicine. Chinese medicine has very effective yang supplementing ingredients to treat kidney yang vacuity cold uterus and also very effective warming ingredients to treat replete cold. Moxibustion, which is the burning of Herba Artemisiae Argyii over certain acupuncture points, is also quite effective for treating either replete or vacuity cold. In both cases, normal menstruation can be restored often with only a single month's treatment. And, as long as the woman does not expose herself again to cold and avoids eating or drinking chilled or iced things, this pattern is not prone to frequent relapse.

The incidence of cold uterus infertility is, in my opinion, not as high in the West as it is in China where it is a leading cause of menstrual and reproductive problems. This is because of our universal use of central heating, our high calorie diet, warm clothes, and less frequent necessity of laboring outdoors in the freezing cold. However, the incidence of this diagnosis in the West does depend upon geographic location. It is more prevalent in colder, damper climates and less prevalent in warmer, drier ones.

Depressive Heat

Depressive heat is usually due to an exacerbation of liver depression qi stagnation. If liver qi becomes excessive and has nowhere to go, it implodes upon itself and transforms into depressive heat. Many Chinese gynecology texts do not list this as a separate pattern of infertility since it is merely a progression of liver qi. Some women will fluctuate between simple liver qi and depressive heat depending upon the season of the year, phase of the moon, phase of their cycle, and their degree of emotional stress. For instance, spring is the season of hyperactivity of the liver during which liver qi often escalates to depressive heat. Likewise, at the full moon and just prior to the onset of menstruation, many women will go from simple liver qi to depressive heat. And extreme, unrelieved stress can cause depressive heat in a person suffering from liver qi at any time.

Just as cold congeals the blood, persistent hat, especially in the liver, eventually either exhausts the blood or makes it run wild. If, because of the liver/spleen disharmony, the spleen's blood transforming function is weak, liver heat will evaporate or exhaust the blood, resulting in scanty, overdue periods. If, on the other hand, a woman's spleen remains robust, this hat may be transferred to the blood while it is stored in the liver and may cause the blood to run recklessly outside its pathways. This then causes excessive bleeding as in abnormally heavy periods, early or too frequent periods, or breakthrough bleeding and spotting. In many cases, there may be liver qi, depressive heat, and blood stasis and, in such cases, there will be bright bleeding but mixed with clots.

Many women with depressive heat may be diagnosed by Western medicine as suffering from various pelvic inflammations and infections, such as PID or salpingitis. However, this heat may be experienced simply as increased irritability, hot flashes, night sweats, palpitations, insomnia, restlessness, a bitter taste in the mouth, and body pain. Besides pain in the pelvis, it can also cause hip and sciatic pain, rib or flank pain, sacroiliac pain, chronic neck and shoulder pain, and headaches and sinusitis, including migraines and cluster headaches. If the heat vents upwards drafting with it the blood, it can cause epistaxis and hemoptysis (nosebleed and coughing blood). If it is mixed with dampness due to simultaneous spleen dysfunction, it can cause thick, white, yellow, or even blood-tinged leukorrhea or vaginal discharge. It may even cause cystitis and kidney stones. The tongue is red or has red rims and there is a scant, typically yellow tongue coating. The pulse is wiry and fast and often fine.

Of the six major Chinese patterns of infertility, women with this pattern tend to have the most and most obvious health complaints. Chinese medicine, both herbs and acupuncture, can usually treat this constellation over a period of several months to a year. These women are usually the most stressed and the most irritable. Therefore, they may tend to be difficult and impatient patients. But, if they understand their disease mechanism and make sincere efforts to modify their lifestyle so it is not so stressful, do daily deep relaxation and every other day aerobic exercise, and are careful to avoid spicy, hot food, fatty, oily foods, coffee, and alcohol, these women's infertility can also be reversed given persistence. When treating this condition, the Chinese style practitioner usually first adjusts the menstrual cycle itself, unless there is some other important complaint, such as hot flashes. Once the period comes on time, is clot free, and of the right volume and duration, the patient's condition has usually gone from depressive heat back to simple liver depression and qi stagnation. This is then addressed until there is no premenstrual breast distention, after which the woman should be fertile.

Phlegm Dampness

I personally have not encountered much phlegm dampness infertility among Western patients. Typically, women with this pattern are obese. In Chinese medicine, excessive adipose tissue is due to excess accumulation of phlegm and dampness due to the spleen not transporting and transforming foods and liquids properly. Instead of separating the pure and turbid of the foods and liquids and sending the pure up to become the qi and blood and the turbid down to become the urine and feces, incompletely combusted and transformed food and fluids condense to form pathogenic dampness and phlegm. These pathologic substances then impede the normal healthy flow of qi and blood. Since dampness is "heavy" and tends to percolate down, just like water through soil, it tends to accumulate in the lower part of the body. This can take the form of edema in the feet and legs, leukorrhea, urinary frequency, dribbling, and incontinence, loose, pasty, sticky stools, mucous mixed in with the stools, lower body obesity, and delayed periods, excessive or scanty periods, or cessation of the periods altogether. The other signs and symptoms of this pattern are excessive sputum or mucous, pallor or puffiness, a heavy feeling of the body, a thin, white or greasy, white tongue coating, a wet or swollen tongue, and a wiry, slippery, or soft pulse.

In the case of phlegm damp infertility, the phlegm and dampness obstruct the flow of qi and blood in the uterus and thus block conception. In addition, since dampness most often originates in the spleen and then impedes spleen function, many women with spleen dampness also suffer from blood vacuity as well. In this case, their period may be late, scant, or absent in part due to insufficient blood to have a regular period. These women will have a pale tongue and a soft, deep, and fine pulse rather than the textbook slippery pulse. However, few of my patients are obese. Rather, my typical female infertility patient is a career woman in her late thirties of relatively normal build. Therefore, I have seldom made a diagnosis of phlegm damp infertility here in the West.

On the other hand, we have seen how dampness can complicate liver qi scenarios due to spleen vacuity and also how dampness can complicate cold disorders, whether vacuity or repletion. It is also common to find phlegm mixed with depressive heat in Western women due to long-term liver qi causing spleen dampness and then the liver qi transforming into depressive heat. In this case, often the liver heat drafts the dampness upwards, causing sinusitis in some and chronic tracheitis in others. Many Western women with over-heated livers experience chronic or recurrent sore throats with the sensation of a glob of mucous stuck in the back of their throats. This is called in Chinese medicine plum seed qi or the feeling as if one had a plum pit stuck in their throat. This can be subdivided into hot and cold plum seed qi. The cold kind is just dampness and cold phlegm which has been drafted up to the throat by a hyperactive liver. The hot kind is composed of hot phlegm drafted up to the throat by depressive heat. Plum seed qi is, interestingly, called neurotic esophageal stenosis in Western medicine which recognizes this as a stress-induced symptom, although it then discounts this symptom as being "just" in the patient's head. Therefore, although I seldom make a diagnosis of simple phlegm dampness amongst my female American patients, phlegm and dampness do often play a part in the typically complicated patterns American patients present.

When phlegm and dampness are a part of a woman's over-all Chinese diagnosis, diet and exercise become all the more important. Exercise mobilizes this dampness and phlegm and either helps to transform or excrete it from the body. Although women who are damp will feel naturally heavy and lethargic, they must be encouraged to become more active and to get more exercise. Once such patients do exercise more, they immediately feel a great improvement. Therefore, exercise must be stressed in such cases. Likewise, diet is of paramount importance since dampness and phlegm are generated by eating too much sugar, dairy, fruit juices, liquids with meals, cold, raw, and greasy, oily foods. Rather, the emphasis should be on cooked, easily digestible foods and primarily vegetables and grains. It is also important such women not over-eat nor drink too much liquid.

Paradoxically, persons with spleen dampness are often thirsty and, therefore, have a tendency to drink too much. This thirst, however, is not a true or healthy thirst. Rather it is due to the fluids ingested being stuck in the spleen which fails to distribute them properly to the rest of the body. The body then registers thirst since it is not getting the benefit of the fluids drunk. So one drinks even more fluids and makes the situation only worse. What is necessary is to reduce fluid intake, especially with meals. This will result in extreme thirst for several days which is necessary if the spleen is to be enabled to process the water in which it is already awash. It is as if the spleen were water-logged and needed to be dried out. A tea-cup of warm, boiled water benefits the digestion when drunk with meals. But an eight ounce glass of something deliciously chilled is a disaster for digestion when poured down over a meal.

Chinese medicine says that dampness is recalcitrant or slow to respond to treatment and that is true. Dampness is not resolved over night. But persistent, regular aerobic exercise, right diet, and Chinese herbs and acupuncture can, over time, rectify this imbalance.

Although there are six basic Chinese patterns of disharmony accounting for female infertility, my experience in treating Western women is that the majority of my patients have a combination of liver depression and qi stagnation, spleen vacuity and/or dampness, blood vacuity, blood stasis, and, from time to time, depressive heat. In addition, most women with infertility who are older than 35 commonly have some combination of the previous Chinese disease mechanisms plus kidney yang vacuity. This kidney yang vacuity is due to the aging process. This kidney yang vacuity is rarely encountered without simultaneous spleen qi vacuity. Yang vacuity can then cause vacuity cold in the uterus which causes or aggravates blood stasis in the uterus.

These women have as an almost universal part of their medical histories the use of oral contraceptives, one or more abortions, some pelvic or lower abdominal inflammation treated with antibiotics, such as cystitis, trichomonas, gonorrhea, or perhaps herpes genitalia, multiple sexual partners since their teens with relatively recent first or second marriages, and current high levels of job, relationship, and survival stress. All these factors have played their part when now these women settle down and choose to become a mother. As the current saying goes, their biological clock is running out and there is a certain sense of hurried desperation in their plight. Each menstrual cycle is an emotional roller-coaster. Each month the woman hopes she is pregnant from mid-cycle until menstruation. As premenstrual signs and symptoms appear, she often becomes depressed at the prospect of losing another month as day by inexorable day she ages. Then, when the period comes, depression, frustration, guilt, and even a sense of failure may set in which may continue even into the next menstrual cycle.

This emotional roller-coaster is a sure-fire formula for aggravating live depression and qi stagnation or for transforming it into depressive heat. And this is why the treatment of modern infertility is often so frustrating. This negative emotional cycle directly perpetuates and worsens the energetic process which is responsible for most Western women's infertility in the first place. In fact, one of my reasons for writing this book is to try to provide information which can help explain this loop and, therefore, help women to disconnect themselves from it. As I have said above under liver qi, women should undergo traditional Chinese medical therapy *first and foremost* simply to be more healthy themselves. Fertility is the natural expression of a body full of life force and blood which is flowing freely and unobstructed. When a woman's signs and symptoms all revert to a more normal range, then the woman is likely to become pregnant.

Therefore, women trying to conceive should place their attention on regulating their menstruation, eliminating premenstrual breast tenderness and any other premenstrual signs and symptoms, and generally improving their health and physical and mental well-being as much as possible. That means they should seek treatment for menoxenia or any menstrual abnormality, any digestive dysfunction, any problem with elimination or perspiration, any problem with appetite, sleep, energy, or mood. In Chinese medicine, when a female patient's period is on time, painless, without particular premenstrual signs and symptoms, is of a sufficient volume and duration, is healthy red color, and is free from clots, when her digestion and elimination are good, energy good, sleep peaceful and sound, and appetite and mood are all good, then this woman is healthy and, if she has not reached menopause, she should be able to conceive.

Many women come to me saying that they have been through the full battery of modern tests and procedures and Western medicine cannot find anything wrong with them. But Chinese medicine pays close attention to small signs and symptoms Western medicine is too quick in dismissing because it has no holistic theory according to which these signs and symptoms are meaningful. Chinese medicine does posit a healthy norm for each and every life function and deviation from this norm suggests a person whose metabolism is out of balance. Since every part and function of the body is inter-related according to Chinese medicine, the Chinese style practitioner assesses the entire individual and does not isolate infertility from the digestion, circulation, one's mood, or diet. Therefore, in ten years of practicing traditional Chinese medicine, I have only seen one woman who complained of infertility who I could not diagnose as suffering from one or more of the above discussed six Chinese disease mechanisms for infertility. In this woman's case, her husband was more likely to be the problem. Otherwise, every infertile American woman I have seen has exhibited signs and symptoms pertaining to one or more of the above six patterns of disharmony.

That means that each woman, according to Chinese medicine, was not only infertile but also *incipiently ill*. Chinese medicine has for over two thousand years placed pre-eminent importance on the prevention of disease before symptomology becomes overt. While infertility may be a woman's primary subjective complaint, the complications of liver qi typically lead to uterine tumors, cervical dysplasia, breast disease, both benign and malignant, hypertension, stroke, heart attack, and cancer. Therefore, there is plenty of good reason for treating liver qi and all its ramifications or any of the above patterns of disharmony regardless of whether one wants to be a mother or not. Each of the above six patterns, if left untreated, can eventually lead to life-threatening disease.

Paradoxically, the best and quickest way for a Western woman in her late thirties to treat her infertility is to de-emphasize her fixation on conceiving and rather emphasize achieving her own personal, vibrant, good health. This is why I often suggest women not to even try to conceive until their menstrual and other related signs and symptoms turn positive. If professional Chinese medicine is combined with right exercise, diet, relaxation, and stress reduction, these goals can usually be achieved in from three to six months or in not more than a year. However, when women try to do Chinese therapy and at the same time ride the infertility emotional roller-coaster each month, therapy drags on and on with no conclusive result. Therefore, before commencing the traditional Chinese medical treatment for infertility, the Western woman should mentally commit herself as whole-heartedly as possible to the *process* as opposed to the product and for a generous period of time.

The worry is, however, that if Chinese medicine does not work, the woman has squandered another irreplaceable six months or a year. This why many women resort to shotgun therapy and a mix and match, eclectic, grab-bag approach. However, we all must make choices in our life which have life and death consequences. My experience is that, usually, we only make our situation even worse when we waffle this way and that, refusing to commit ourselves to a single line of action. If I were promoting some new, personal concoction of my own, a certain skepticism would be healthy on the part of my patients. But Chinese medicine is no shot in the dark. Rather, it is the oldest, continually practiced, literate, professional medicine in the world. Its methods, although not yet well-known here in the West, have been time-tested over two millennia. This treatment is hardly experimental and it works here in the West just as it works in the Peoples' Republic of China.

There are a few differences between the treatment of infertility here in the West and in China. In China, woman marry in their early twenties one year out of college. Therefore, women diagnosed as being infertile in China are usually in their mid to late twenties and there is not the same sense of hurry-up desperation. Secondly, there is far, far less stress in China than here in the West. The pace is much slower and gentler and most of life is a given. We have paid a very high price for our affluence, our freedom, and our mobility. Because there is less stress in general in China, Chinese clinicians see a much broader range of cases of infertility. Whereas here in the West, there definitely are certain common reasons why women of a certain age and socio-economic group are experiencing a higher than normal incidence of infertility. And third, Chinese medicine in China is an accepted and time-honored health option. It is the other great medical system available in China (besides Western medicine) and Chinese patients opting for traditional Chinese medical treatment understand its methodology and terminology better than do Western patients. Therefore, they are more willing to persevere with Chinese medicine longer and more whole-heartedly.

However, except for these few differences, traditional Chinese medicine is just as practical and effective here in the West as in the Far East. Chinese medicine can accurately diagnose and treat the patterns of infertility Western women present as the following case histories show.

Case Histories

Case I: This patient was 40 years old when she first visited me. Her main complaint was infertility. She had been married for ten years or so and had conceived only once three years previously when she had had a miscarriage. Her Western doctors had not found any particular organic problems. She had taken Prednisone for two and a half years for antibodies found in her blood to her husband's sperm. After one year, her sperm antibody test turned negative. Currently the woman was taking chlomiphene, a common Western fertility drug.

Prior to the miscarriage, her period had come at 28 days with severe cramps. One MD had diagnosed endometriosis. After the miscarriage, her cycle lengthened to 31 days, until beginning chlomiphene when it began coming on the 26th day. Since the miscarriage, her cramps were mild with a small to moderate flow lasting three to four days. Her menstruate was dark but not very dark and contained occasional clots. Her tongue was pale and fluted with a normal, thin, white coating. Her pulse was wiry with a tendency towards being fast. The patient had variable premenstrual breast distention and sighed frequently during her initial visit.

Her Chinese medical diagnosis was liver qi with depressive heat. Her wiry pulse indicated the liver qi, as did the darkish blood, breast distention, and sighing. Her pale, fluted tongue suggested some blood vacuity due to spleen vacuity in turn due to liver invading the spleen. And her slightly but none the less early period and fastish pulse suggested the depressive heat which is common in women with liver qi in their late thirties and throughout their forties. Because it seemed such an uncomplicated case by Chinese standards, I simply prescribed a modification of Free and Easy Powder to be taken in decoction beginning at mid-cycle and continued through the onset of her period. The patient was also advised on deep relaxation, aerobic exercise, and dietary modifications which she readily accepted.

Four months later, this woman was pregnant after three months of Chinese herbal medicine. At four and a half weeks of pregnancy, I treated her again with Chinese herbs for morning sickness due to liver invading the stomach. Within six days her nausea was under control. Since qi vacuity is the single most common cause of miscarriage according to Chinese medicine and since qi is manufactured by the spleen/stomach through the process of digestion,

Chinese doctors feel it is very important preventively to treat morning sickness and there are effective herbal and acupuncture treatments for it. One week before her expected due date, I prescribed an herbal formula to help relax her liver so she would have a quicker, less painful labor and a few days after her due date she gave birth to a healthy baby boy.

Case II: This woman was 36 year old. Her major complaint was infertility. Her chiropractor had diagnosed her as having a tipped uterus. She was constipated quite often and x-rays showed that her intestines "looped too much". She had never had a normal menstrual cycle except on birth control pills which she used for 10 years beginning at age 22. Otherwise, her periods tended to be delayed, coming every two to three months. Usually she had a scant flow which was darkish brown. She had shoulder and neck tension and was 10 pounds over-weight. Her tongue coating was normal but the tongue itself was a little dark. Her liver pulse was quite strong and wiry, but the pulses corresponding to her pelvis were very sunken. Abdominal palpation showed that she was very sensitive around her belly button and her lower left abdomen. An endometrial biopsy suggested that she was not producing enough progesterone to facilitate implantation.

My Chinese diagnosis was infertility and delayed menstruation due to stagnant qi and blood stasis which was revealed primarily in her pulse. The strong, wiry pulse in her liver position meant liver depression and the sunken pulse in her pelvic positions indicated blood stasis. This then resulted in impeded or delayed menstruation and constipation. Otherwise, the patient was relatively quite healthy. I prescribed a Chinese herbal formula for her to take daily and taught her how to do moxibustion on herself in order to rectify the position of her uterus. This she did every other day for one week. After a week, her chiropractor pronounced here uterus was now in its proper place. This was attended by alleviation of her long-term constipation and her next period came at 38 days. In addition, her neck and shoulder pain were much improved. This shows how the entire body is an inter-related, functional unit and how traditional Chinese medicine treats the entire person.

The patient continued taking Chinese herbs for another three months at which point she conceived, but she miscarried at her twelfth week of pregnancy. Unfortunately, this woman lived three hours drive away and I was not able to treat her for threatened abortion. Many women who conceive after being infertile for some time miscarry at first. This is because, in their rush to get pregnant, they have not undergone sufficient Chinese therapy to get their qi in really good order. Therefore, their qi vacuity or some amount of residual stasis and stagnation often causes the miscarriage. In this woman's case, her liver depression transformed into depressive heat. This, combined with the residual blood stasis which had not been completely eliminated, caused her to miscarry.

Her next period came six weeks after the miscarriage. She continued to take qi-regulating and blood-quickening Chinese herbs. Her bowel movements continued to be regular and her periods came on time. Her menstruate became fuller and less dark. After about another six months of taking Chinese herbs, this woman conceived and carried this child to full term. Eventually she gave birth without problem to a healthy little girl.

For further and more up to date medical diagnosis and treatment of female infertility, see Bob Flaws's *Fulfilling the Essence: A Handbook of Traditional & Contemporary Chinese Treatments for Female Infertility*. Blue Poppy Press, 1993.

FINDING A PRACTITIONER OF TRADITIONAL CHINESE MEDICINE

Traditional Chinese medicine is a rapidly rising star within the Western alternative health care community. As of this writing, there are more than 50 American schools and colleges of acupuncture and Chinese medicine. That means that the number of professional American practitioners of this art is growing by about 1,000 new practitioners per year. Many American practitioners have also either gone to medical school in Asia or have gone to Asia for post-graduate training. And, of course, many Asian doctors have immigrated to the United States in the last twenty years.

In addition, in the U.S., there is a National Council of Acupuncture Schools and Colleges which helps to over-see and regulate the quality of training and education, a National Commission for the Certification of Acupuncturists which helps to insure minimum, entry level, professional competence, and various state and national professional associations, such as the American Association of Acupuncture and Oriental Medicine and the National Acupuncture & Oriental Medicine Alliance, which help to regulate professional ethics, network amongst practitioners, and provide continuing, post-graduate education. Acupuncture has now been legalized as a state-approved health care modality in over a score of states and in many others, favorable legislation is in the process of being enacted.

In states where acupuncture is licensed and state regulated, one should be able to find the names of local practitioners in the yellow pages of their phone book or by contacting their state Department of Health, Board of Medical Examiners, or Department of Regulatory Agencies. In such states, it is wise to insure that potential practitioners are, in fact, state licensed. In states without licensure, it is best to seek out those practitioners who are nationally board certified. Such practitioners typically append the initials Dipl. Ac., for Diplomate of Acupuncture, after their names. These national board exams insure minimal professional competency and not less than the equivalent of two full years of academic and clinical training specifically in acupuncture.

In the United States, not all acupuncturists are practitioners of Chinese herbal medicine, but almost without exception, all American practitioners of Chinese herbal medicine are also acupuncturists. As yet, only a handful of states include Chinese herbal education and examination in their licensing and, until now, there is no national herbal board exam. Therefore, it is important to query potential practitioners on the school, nature, and extent of their Chinese herbal training. In general, the practice of Chinese Internal or herbal medicine is more demanding and requires more education and experience than the practice of acupuncture. The NCCA now does offer a national certification exam in Chinese herbal medicine. Successful graduates of this exam append the letters Dipl.C.H., standing for Diplomate of Chinese Herbs, after their names.

When searching out a qualified and knowledgeable practitioner, satisfied, word of mouth referrals are important. Therefore, it is also appropriate to ask for references from previous patients treated for the same problem. Likewise, it is important that the practitioner be able to communicate with the patient in order to explain their Chinese diagnosis and the rationale behind their treatment plan. In all cases, a professional practitioner of Chinese medicine should be able and willing to give a written traditional Chinese diagnosis of the patient's case. Also, I personally suggest that patients select practitioners who belong to both local and national Chinese medicine/acupuncture professional associations. Such associations offer referrals of professional members in good standing and high repute. In addition, such associations almost always have a code of professional ethics which their members promise to uphold and this further insures the quality and professionalism of the care they provide.

Traditional Chinese medicine, including acupuncture, is a discrete and independent health care profession. It is not a technique to be added to the bag of tricks of some other profession. It takes just as long *or longer* to learn Chinese medicine and acupuncture as it does to learn allopathy, chiropractic, naturopathy, or homeopathy, and previous training in one of these systems in no way confers *a priori* competence or knowledge in Chinese medicine or acupuncture. Therefore, I heartily advise prospective patients seeking to avail themselves of the benefits of traditional Chinese medicine to seek out professionally trained practitioners of this system. As suggested above under acupuncture and endometriosis, just as one would not hire a plumber to do electrical wiring, so patients should receive Chinese medicine from professionally trained practitioners of Chinese medicine.

For further information regarding the American practice of Chinese medicine and acupuncture and for referrals to local professional associations and practitioners, prospective patients may contact:

American Association of Acupuncture and Oriental Medicine
433 Front St.
Catasauqua, PA 18032-2506
(610) 433-2448

National Commission for the Certification of Acupuncturists
P.O. Box 97075
Washington, DC 20090-7075
(202) 232-1404

National Acupuncture & Oriental Medicine Alliance
PO Box 77511
Seattle, WA 98177-3511
(206) 524-3511

CONCLUSION

The purpose of writing this book has been to share with Western women the knowledge that traditional Chinese medicine can effectively and cost-efficiently treat and cure both endometriosis and infertility. It is my hope that if more women knew about the effectiveness of traditional Chinese medicine in treating these two conditions, more women would seek out and begin Chinese style treatment as a *first option* early on when their condition is still relatively simple and easy to remedy. This could save a great deal of both physical and emotional pain for Western women who are already under such great personal and societal stress.

Secondly, if more women experienced the effectiveness of traditional Chinese medicine in dealing with these two specific conditions, then more people in the West would be exposed to the fact that Chinese medicine is a generally effective alternative and complement to modern Western medicine. These same women would be all the more likely to seek traditional Chinese health care for other illnesses and complaints as would their friends and relatives. This would then help to popularize the use of traditional Chinese medicine in this country in general, which, I believe, would be a great boon for the health of people in the developed nations.

And third, it has been my intention in writing this book to share with everyone the rational and holistic vision of Chinese medicine. Traditional Chinese medicine is not just a collection of exotic and outlandish, empirical therapies. Rather, its greatest treasure is its humane and rational explanation of why and how we as humans living in this world get sick the way we do. Chinese medicine offers us the opportunity to take responsibility for and to regain control over our own health and well-being. Ultimately, it is a blueprint for living a healthy, sane, and harmonious life.

ENDOMETRIOSIS, INFERTILITY AND TRADITIONAL CHINESE MEDICINE: A Laywoman's Guide by Bob Flaws ISBN 0-936185-14-7 $9.95

THE BREAST CONNECTION: A Laywoman's Guide to the Treatment of Breast Disease by Chinese Medicine
by Honora Lee Wolfe ISBN 0-936185-61-9, $9.95

NINE OUNCES: A Nine Part Program For The Prevention of AIDS in HIV Positive Persons by Bob Flaws ISBN 0-936185-12-0 $9.95

THE TREATMENT OF CANCER BY INTEGRATED CHINESE-WESTERN MEDICINE by Zhang Dai-zhao, trans. by Zhang Ting-liang & Bob Flaws, ISBN 0-936185-11-2, $18.95

A HANDBOOK OF TRADITIONAL CHINESE DERMATOLOGY by Liang Jian-hui, trans. by Zhang Ting-liang & Bob Flaws, ISBN 0-936185-07-4 $15.95

A HANDBOOK OF TRADITIONAL CHINESE GYNECOLOGY by Zhejiang College of TCM, trans. by Zhang Ting-liang, ISBN 0-936185-06-6 (4nd edit.) $22.95

PRINCE WEN HUI'S COOK: Chinese Dietary Therapy by Bob Flaws & Honora Lee Wolfe, ISBN 0-912111-05-4, $12.95 (Published by Paradigm Press, Brookline, MA)

THE DAO OF INCREASING LONGEVITY AND CONSERVING ONE'S LIFE by Anna Lin & Bob Flaws, ISBN 0-936185-24-4 $16.95

FIRE IN THE VALLEY: The TCM Diagnosis and Treatment of Vaginal Diseases by Bob Flaws ISBN 0-936185-25-2 $16.95

HIGHLIGHTS OF ANCIENT ACUPUNCTURE PRESCRIPTIONS trans. by Honora Lee Wolfe & Rose Crescenz ISBN 0-936185-23-6, $14.95

ARISAL OF THE CLEAR: A Simple Guide to Healthy Eating According to Traditional Chinese Medicine by Bob Flaws, ISBN #-936185-27-9 $8.95

PEDIATRIC BRONCHITIS: Its Cause, Diagnosis & Treatment According to Traditional Chinese Medicine trans. by Gao Yu-li and Bob Flaws, ISBN 0-936185-26-0 $15.95

AIDS & ITS TREATMENT ACCORDING TO TRADITIONAL CHINESE MEDICINE by Huang Bing-shan, trans. by Fu-Di & Bob Flaws, ISBN 0-936185-28-7 $24.95

ACUTE ABDOMINAL SYNDROMES: Their. Diagnosis & Treatment by Combined Chinese-Western Medicine by Alon Marcus, ISBN 0-936185-31-7 $16.95

MY SISTER, THE MOON: The Diagnosis & Treatment of Menstrual Diseases by Traditional Chinese Medicine by Bob Flaws, ISBN 0-936185-34-1, $24.95

FU QING-ZHU'S GYNECOLOGY trans. by Yang Shou-zhong and Liu Da-wei, ISBN 0-936185-35-X, $22.95

FLESHING OUT THE BONES: The Importance of Case Histories in Chinese Medicine trans. by Charles Chace. ISBN 0-936185-30-9, $18.95

CLASSICAL MOXIBUSTION SKILLS in Contemporary Clinical Practice by Sung Baek, ISBN 0-936185-16-3 $12.95

THE MEDICAL I CHING: Oracle of the Healer Within by Miki Shima, OMD, ISBN 0-936185-38-4, $19.95

MASTER TONG'S ACUPUNC-TURE: An Ancient Lineage for Modern Practice, trans. and commentary by Miriam Lee, OMD, ISBN 0-936185-37-6, $19.95

A HANDBOOK OF TCM UROL-OGY & MALE SEXUAL DYSFUNCTION by Anna Lin, OMD, ISBN 0-936185-36-8, $16.95

MASTER HUA'S CLASSIC OF THE CENTRAL VISCERA by Hua Tuo, ISBN 0-936185-43-0, $21.95

THE HEART & ESSENCE OF DAN-XI'S METHODS OF TREATMENT by Xu Dan-xi, trans. by Yang Shou-zhong, ISBN 0-926185-49-X, $21.95

STATEMENTS OF FACT IN TRA-DITIONAL CHINESE MEDICINE by Bob Flaws, ISBN 0-936185-52-X, $12.95

IMPERIAL SECRETS OF HEALTH & LONGEVITY by Bob Flaws, ISBN 0-936185-51-1, $9.95

THE SYSTEMATIC CLASSIC OF ACUPUNCTURE & MOXIBUSTION (*Jia Yi Jing*) by Huang-fu Mi, trans. by Yang Shou-zhong and Charles Chace, ISBN 0-936185-29-5, $79.95

CHINESE MEDICINAL WINES & ELIXIRS by Bob Flaws, ISBN 0-936185-58-9, $18.95

THE DIVINELY RESPONDING CLASSIC: A Translation of the *Shen Ying Jing* **from** *Zhen Jiu Da Cheng*, trans. by Yang Shou-zhong & Liu Feng-ting ISBN 0-936185-55-4, $15.95

PAO ZHI: An Introduction to Processing Chinese Medicinals to Enhance Their Therapeutic Effect, by Philippe Sionneau, ISBN 0-936185-62-1, $34.95

THE BOOK OF JOOK: Chinese Medic-inal Porridges, An Alternative to the Typi-cal Western Breakfast, by Bob Flaws, ISBN0-936185-60-0, $16.95

SHAOLIN SECRET FORMULAS for the Treatment of External Injuries, by De Chan, ISBN 0-936185-08-2, $18.95

AGING & BLOOD STASIS: A New Approach to TCM Geriatrics, by Yan De-xin, ISBN 0-936185-63-5, $21.95

CHINESE MEDICAL PALMISTRY: Your Health in Your Hand, by Zong Xiao-fan & Gary Liscum, ISBN 0-936185-64-3, $15.95

THE SECRET OF CHINESE PULSE DIAGNOSIS by Bob Flaws, ISBN 0-936185-67-8, $17.95

LOW BACK PAIN: Care & Preven-tion with Traditional Chinese Medicine by Douglas Frank, ISBN 0-936185-66-X, $9.95

A COMPENDIUM OF TCM PAT-TERNS & TREATMENTS by Bob Flaws & Daniel Finney, ISBN 0-936185-70-8, $29.95

**ACUPUNCTURE AND MOXIBUS-
TION FORMULAS & TREATMENTS**
by Cheng Dan-an, trans. By Wu Ming, ISBN
0-936185-68-6, $22.95

**THE TREATMENT OF DISEASE IN
TCM, Vol I: Diseases of the Head &
Face Including Mental/Emotional Dis-
orders** by Philippe Sionneau & Lü Gang,
ISBN 0-936185-69-4, $21.95

**THE TREATMENT OF DISEASE IN
TCM, Vol. II: Diseases of the Eyes,
Ears, Nose, & Throat** by Philippe
Sionneau & Lü Gang, ISBN 0-936185-69-4,
$21.95

**KEEPING YOUR CHILD HEALTHY
WITH CHINESE MEDICINE: A Par-
ent's Guide to the Care & Prevention of
Common Childhood Diseases**, by Bob
Flaws, ISBN 0-936185-71-6, $15.95

**CHINESE MEDICINAL TEAS: Sim-
ple, Proven, Folk Formulas for Common Diseases & Promoting Health**, by
Zong Xiao-fan & Gary Liscum, ISBN 0-
936185-76-7, $19.95